The Illustrated Dictionary of Pregnancy and Birth has over 450 entries – from Alphafetoprotein to Old Wives' Tales; Apgar Test to Maternity Leave; Braxton-Hicks Contractions to Zygote; Dental Checks to Vernix – and many clear and helpful illustrations. Comprehensive and straightforward, it includes everything you'll need to know for a happy, healthy pregnancy and birth.

Heather Welford is a mother, and freelance journalist specialising in the areas of pregnancy, health and child care. She writes regularly for Parents magazine. She has called on experience and research, and the advice of a leading obstetrician and a midwife to compile all the information both a new or experienced mother could want, in an attractive and accessible format.

THE ILLUSTRATED
DICTIONARY OF PREGNANCY AND BIRTH

THE ILLUSTRATED
DICTIONARY OF PREGNANCY AND BIRTH

HEATHER WELFORD

London
UNWIN PAPERBACKS
Boston   Sydney   Wellington

Publisher's Acknowledgements
Thanks are due to the following for their help with illustrative material. Maggie Raynor, Pete and Jennie Smith for the line drawings. Nicola Blakeney, Alan Duns, Paul Ostrer, *Petit Format* Picture Agency, *Transworld* Picture Agency and St Bartholomew's Hospital for the use of photographic material.

First published in Great Britain by Allen & Unwin 1986
First published by Unwin Paperbacks 1987

This book is copyright under the Berne Convention.
No reproduction without permission. All rights reserved.

**UNWIN® PAPERBACKS, an imprint of Unwin Hyman Ltd,
40 Museum Street, London WC1A 1LU, UK**

Unwin Paperbacks, an imprint of Unwin Hyman Ltd,
Park Lane, Hemel Hempstead, Herts HP2 4TE

Allen & Unwin Australia Pty Ltd,
8 Napier Street, North Sydney, NSW 2060, Australia

Unwin Paperbacks, A Division of Unwin Hyman Ltd,
with the Port Nicholson Press
PO Box 11-838 Wellington, New Zealand

© Heather Welford 1986, 1987

British Library Cataloguing in Publication Data

Welford, Heather
  The illustrated dictionary of pregnancy and birth
  1. Pregnancy – Dictionaries
  2. Childbirth – Dictionaries
  I. Title
  618.2'03'21   RG524
  ISBN 0-04-612047-5

Photoset in 10½ on 12 point Palatino
by Nene Phototypesetters Ltd, Northampton
and printed at The Bath Press, Avon

To Beth, Tim and Katie

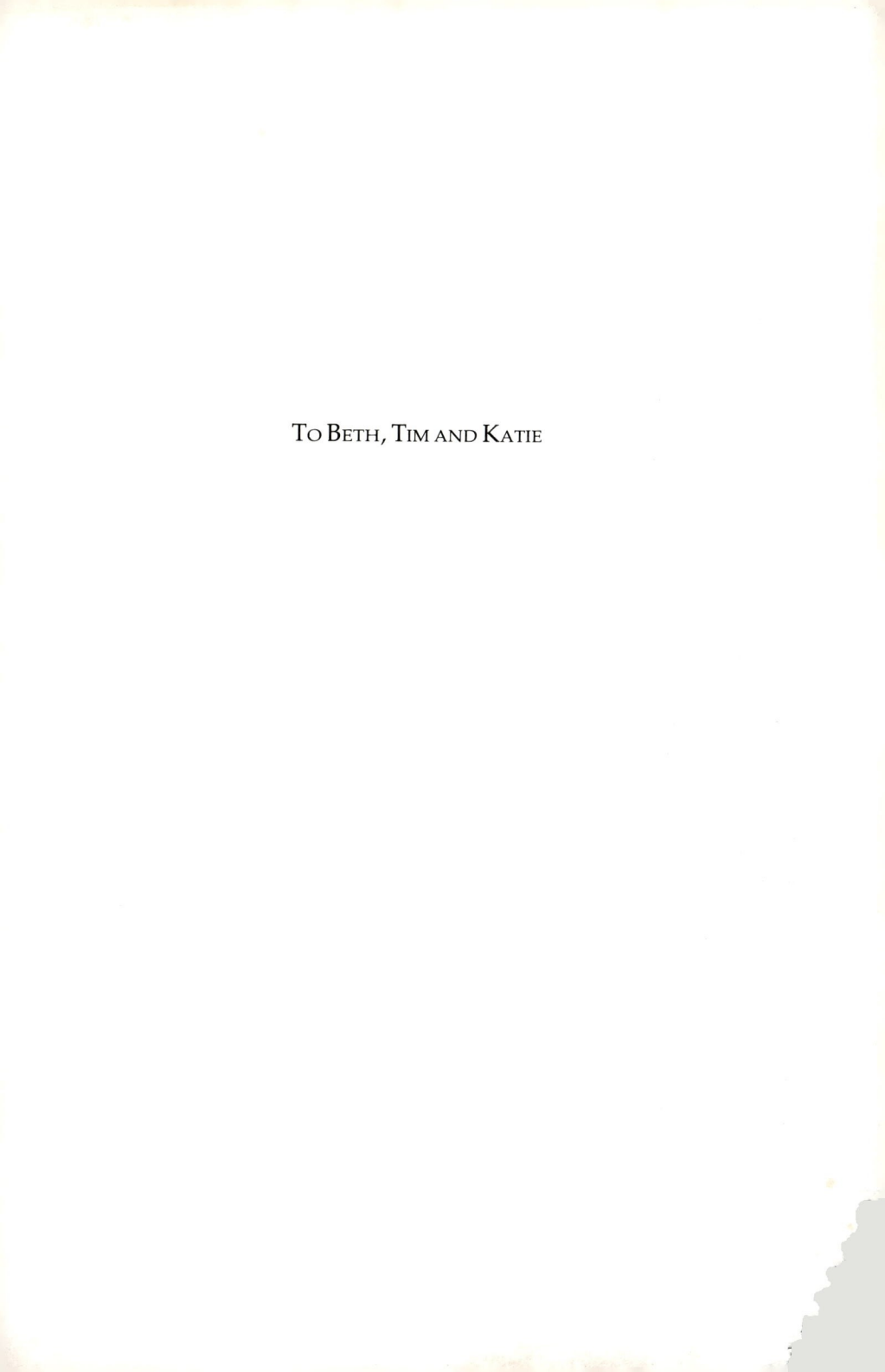

AUTHOR'S NOTE

Certain words in the text are cross-referenced by being printed in italics. This is done when it might be helpful or enlightening for you to look up that particular head-word. It is not done in every case. For instance, you don't need to read the complete entry for caesarean section every time it is mentioned in another context. All topics – including those not used as head-words – are indexed at the back of the book.

Babies, in line with real life, are sometimes 'she' and sometimes 'he'.

CONTENTS

AUTHOR'S ACKNOWLEDGEMENTS
Page xi

INTRODUCTION
Page xiii

LIST OF ENTRIES
Page xv

USEFUL ADDRESSES
Page 135

INDEX
Page 137

AUTHOR'S ACKNOWLEDGMENTS

Many people have helped in the creation of this book. The years I have spent writing for *Parents* magazine have allowed me to share in the wide experience and knowledge of colleagues and contributors. The many thousands of readers' letters to the magazine's 'help' pages have shown me something of what today's parents and parents-to-be want to know. In my personal life, friends and colleagues in the National Childbirth Trust, playgroups and toddler clubs I've been involved in have taught me much about family life today.

Two people in particular, however, helped immeasurably by reading over the manuscript of this book, checking it for accuracy and making their own highly-valued comments. They were Cyril Young, MSc MRCOG, a leading obstetrician and gynaecologist (and father, too), who has also contributed to *Parents* for many years; and mother and midwife Jackie Moore, now working in the community for a northern health authority. My grateful thanks go to both of them, though responsibility for any errors that remain is, of course, my own. In addition, I want to thank both Melissa Brooks who copyedited the manuscript with sensitivity and flair whilst pregnant with her first baby, Chloe, and Bobbie Rolfe, who typed the final manuscript so speedily and efficiently.

Thanks, too, go to my husband Derek Neil, who gave encouragement as well as love . . . as did my three children, though they're too young to know it. My third child was conceived, carried and born during the preparation of the book, which certainly allowed me to keep in touch with the subject matter I was handling. And finally, thanks also to Christine Lees, who looked after my elder two children so happily and so well, twice a week for many months, with my total confidence and trust, allowing me time to complete this project. Christine tragically died in a road accident in August 1986, at the age of 29. Those who knew her remember her with love.

HEATHER WELFORD

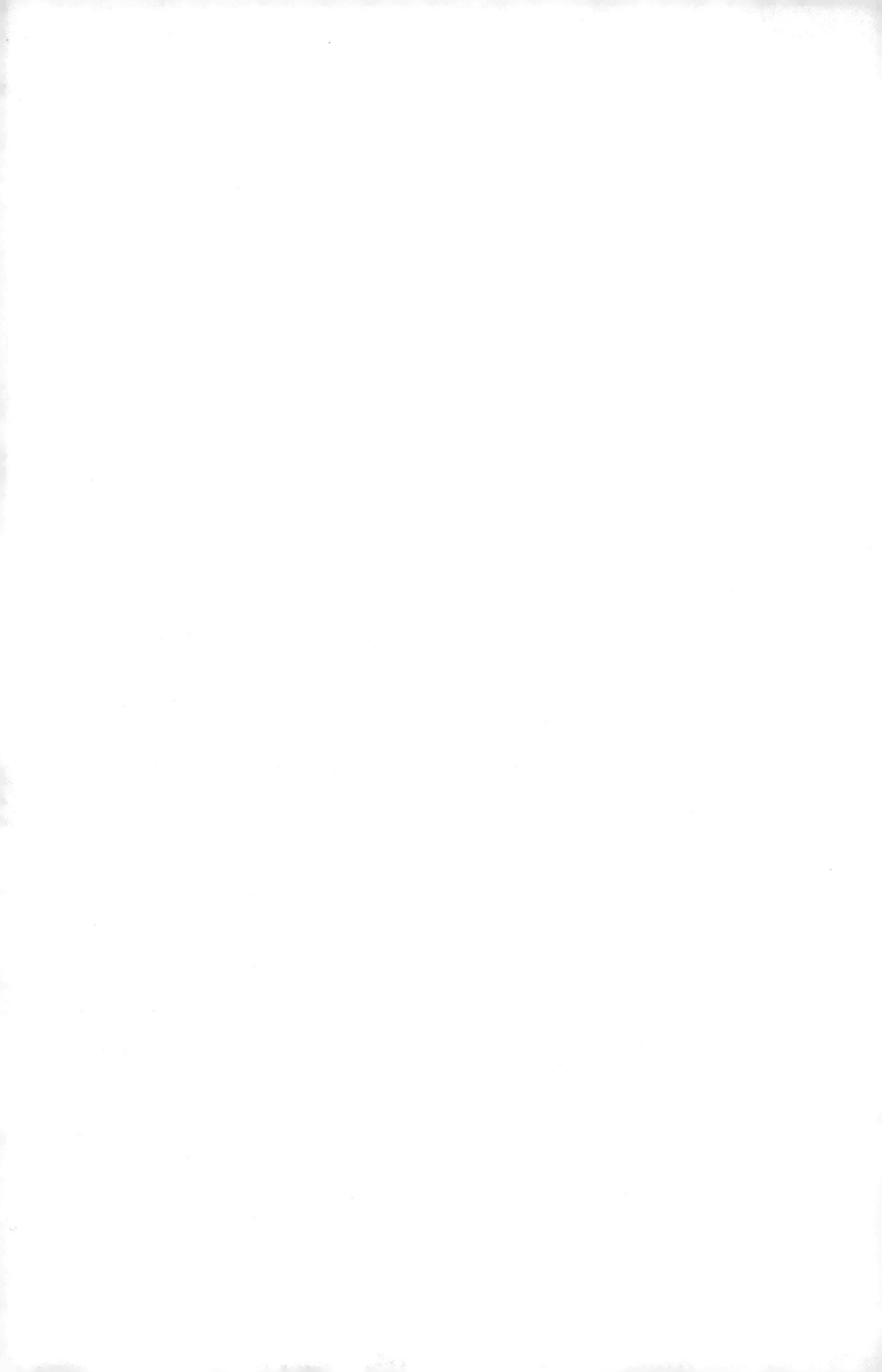

INTRODUCTION

What do today's mothers want from pregnancy and birth? No one can answer that with certainty. Some voices advocate childbirth without drugs; they may campaign for home births; or they may speak out for the merits of delivery in positions quite different from the ones our midwives and doctors are familiar with. All these standpoints, and other similar ones, spring at least partly from a modern-day wish for a more spontaneous, natural way of life. It began in the sixties, with the 'peace and love' message of the young, and continued through to the seventies and eighties, with serious attempts to challenge accepted wisdom about what we eat and the way it affects our health, and about life-style and the authority of the medical profession.

At the same time as all this was going on, however, medical technology made huge advances, and there were large increases in health service spending during the boom years of the early seventies. For the maternity services, this resulted in (among other phenomena) the machinery and specialist knowledge that led to ultrasound scanning, fetal monitoring and epidural anaesthesia becoming almost universally available.

Yet I see no reason for everyone – mothers, midwives, obstetricians, GPs, health service planners – to suddenly start deciding which 'side' they're on. Yes, on the face of it, high-tech obstetrics seems in direct opposition to the movement for drug-free natural childbirth. But it needn't be like this. My experience as a journalist in this field, and as a mother, has convinced me that the greatest need is for the individual woman to be informed, as of right, of the choices available to her, to be treated respectfully, gently and sympathetically throughout pregnancy and labour. Where there are medical problems, doctors need to be prepared to explain the factors leading them to decide on (for example) induction, and to acknowledge that women can, on the whole, accept that clinical decisions aren't always cut-and-dried certainties. More generally, technology needs to be evaluated, its side-effects carefully assessed and all the disadvantages and advantages communicated to mothers. Even apparently simple forms of intervention – such as shaving the pubic hair – have drawbacks that should prevent their widespread or routine use.

Of course, intervention is essential in many births. Many mothers and babies are grateful that the technology and the expertise exist. However, because so many obstetricians disagree so often (not always in public) about its application, the voice of the individual woman needs to be heard, too. Talking with her doctor, her midwife and, yes, her friends and family, listening to informed opinion and making known her own, she can reach the decision that's right for her. She should have confidence that whatever happens during the birth, nothing will cause her to feel guilty or threatened or 'taken over'; she will trust the staff to involve her, to consult her and to do the best for her and her baby.

However, an individual's choice in these matters can be drastically limited if

INTRODUCTION

obstetricians, maternity units or health authorities have rigid policies that decree the availability of home birth, or where staff shortgages mean epidurals can only be given at certain, limited times of the day or night. If we believe in choice, then there's surely no contradiction in calling for 24-hour availability of epidurals in all maternity units, plus health service backing for more home births.

My book has been written firmly from a mother's point of view. I hope you will read it and find out most of what you want to know about your pregnancy, and about what to expect during the birth and the first few weeks with your baby. Perhaps you'll extend your knowledge by reading other books, and by talking to the people around you and to those caring for your health during this time. Then, when it comes to choosing among different options (and I hope you have a choice) you may have the confidence, and the support and help of those whose views you respect, to make up your own mind.

HEATHER WELFORD
October 1986

LIST OF ENTRIES

A

Abdomen
Abortion
Acceleration of Labour
Active Birth
Acupuncture
Adoption
Afterbirth
Afterpains
Age of Mother
AID
AIH
Alcohol
Allergies
All-Fours
Alphafetoprotein (AFP)
Amenorrhoea
Amniocentesis
Amniotic Fluid
Amniotic Sac
Anaemia
Anaesthetist
Analgesia
Anencephaly
Ankles, Swollen
Ante-Natal
Ante-Natal Care
Ante-Natal Classes
Ante-Natal Clinic
Ante-Partum Haemorrhage
Anterior Lip (of Cervix)
Anterior Presentation
Antibodies
Anti-D Gamma Globulin
Anxiety in Labour
Anxiety in Pregnancy
Apgar Test
Apnoea Mattress
Appearance of New Baby
Artificial Rupture of the Membranes

B

Baby Clinic
Backache
Bath in Labour
Bathing Baby
Bearing Down
Bedding for Baby
Bedrest
Bicornuate Uterus
Birth
Birth Certificate
Birth Chair
Birthing Rooms
Birthmarks
Birth Position
Bladder
Blastocyst
Bleeding
Blighted Ovum
Blocked Ducts
Blood Pressure
Blood Tests
Blood Transfusion
Bloom of Pregnancy
Bonding
Booking Appointment
Bottle Feeding
Bras
Braxton-Hicks Contractions
Breastfeeding
Breast Milk
Breast Pumps
Breasts
Breast Shells
Breathing
Breathing Difficulties
Breathlessness
Breech Presentation
Brow Presentation
Butterfly Mask

C

Caesarean Section
Calcium
Caput
Carpal Tunnel Syndrome
Cartiocography
Castor Oil
Catheter
Caul
Cephalhaematoma
Cephalic
Cervical Erosion
Cervical Smear Test
Cervix
Child Benefit
Chloasma
Choosing a Hospital
Chorion Villus Sampling
Chorionic Gonadotrophin
Chromosome
Circumcision
Cleft Lip/Palate
Clothes for Baby
Clothes for Mother
Colostrum
Community Health Council
Community Midwife
Complications of Pregnancy

LIST OF ENTRIES

Conception
Confinement
Congenital
Congenital Dislocation of the Hip
Constipation
Consultant
Contraception
Contractions
Convulsions
Co-operation Card
Corpus Luteum
Cramp
Crowning
Crying Baby
Cyst
Cystitis
Cutting the Cord

D

D & C
Dangers to avoid
Dating the Pregnancy
Death in Childbirth
Decidua
Deep Transverse Arrest
Delivery Room
Dental Checks
Development of Fetus
Diabetes
Diaphragm
Diaphragm (contraceptive cap)
Diarrhoea
Diet
Dilatation
Dilatation and Curettage
Discharge
Discharge from Hospital
Disproportion
Diuretics
Domino Scheme
Double Uterus
Doula
Down's Syndrome
Drip
Drugs

E

Eating in Labour
Eclampsia
Ectopic Pregnancy
EDD/EDC
Effacement
Embryo
Emergency Birth
Emergency Caesarean Section
Emergencies in Labour
Emergencies in Pregnancy
Emotions after the Birth
Emotions during Pregnancy
Endometrium
Enema
Energy Spurt
Engagement of Head
Engorgement of Breasts
Entonox
Epidural Anaesthesia
Episiotomy
Equipment for Baby
Exercise in Pregnancy
Expressing Milk

F

Face Presentation
Fallopian Tubes
False Labour
False Pregnancy
Family Doctor
Family Medical History
Family Planning
Fathers
Fear of Childbirth
Feeding
Fertilisation
Fetal Distress
Fetal Monitor
Fetal Movements
Fetus
Fibre in Diet
First Feed
First Stage of Labour
Flat Babies
Flat Nipples

Fluid Retention
Folic Acid
Fontanelle
Forceps
Forewaters
Friends
FSH
Fundus

G

Gammaglobulin
Gas and Air
Gene
General Anaesthetic
Genetic Counselling
German Measles
Glucose/Dextrose Drip
GP
GP Unit
Guthrie Test
Gynaecologist

H

Habitual Abortion
Haemoglobin
Haemorrhage
Hair in Pregnancy
Handicap
HCG
Head of Baby
Headaches
Health before Pregnancy
Health during Pregnancy
Health Visitor
Heartburn
Heart of Fetus
Height of Mother
Herpes
High Risk
High Tech
Home Birth
Home Help
Hormones
Hospital Birth
Hospital Discharge
Hospital Gown
Hospital Nursery

LIST OF ENTRIES

Hospital Staff
Hydatidiform Mole
Hydrocephaly/
 Hydrocephalus
Hygiene
Hypertension
Hyperventilation
Hypnosis
Hypoglycaemia
Hypospadias

I

Incompetent Cervix
Incomplete Abortion
Incubator
Induction
Infertility
Insomnia
Intensive Care
Intercourse
Internal Examination
Intra-Uterine Death
Inverted Nipples
Involution of Uterus
Iron
Itching in Pregnancy

J

Jaundice

K

Ketones
Kick Chart

L

Labour
Labour Companion
Labour Ward
Lactation
Lanugo
Latching On
Leboyer, Frederic
Length of Labour
Let-Down Reflex

LH
Lie of Baby in Uterus
Lightening
Light-for-Dates
Linea Nigra
Liquor
Lithotomy Position
Lochia
Low-Lying Placenta

M

Manual Removal of the
 Placenta
Massage
Mastitis
Maternity Leave
Maternity Rights
Maternity Wear
Meconium
Medical History
Membranes
Midwife
Milk Banks
Miscarriage
Monitor
Montgomery's Tubercles
Morning Sickness
Moulding
Movement in Labour
Mucus Extraction
Mucus Plug
Multigravida
Multipara
Multiple Pregnancy

N

N.A.D.
Nappies
Nappy Changing
Natural Childbirth
Nausea
Navel
Neural Tube Defects
Nipple Shield
Notes

O

Observations in Labour
Obstetrician
Occipito Posterior
Occiput
Oedema
Oestriol
Oestriol Tests
Oestrogens
Old Wives' Tales
Operculum
Orgasm
Os
Ovulation
Oxygen
Oxytocin

P

Pain in Labour
Pain Relief
Palpation
Panting in Labour
Parentcraft Classes
Paternity Leave
Pelvic Floor Exercises
Peri-Natal
Peri-Natal Death
Perineum
Pessaries
Pethidine
Phantom Pregnancy
Phenylketonuria
Piles
Pill, The
Placenta
Placenta Praevia
Placental Abruption
Placental Insufficiency
Polyhydramnios
Positions for the First Stage
Positions for the Second
 Stage
Posterior Presentation
Post-Mature
Post-Natal
Post-Natal Blues
Post-Natal Depression
Post-Natal Examination

xvii

LIST OF ENTRIES

Post-Natal Exercises
Post-Partum Haemorrhage
Pre-Eclampsia
Pregnancy
Prepping
Pre-Term Baby
Primigravida
Primipara
Progesterone
Prolactin
Prolapse
Prolapse of the Cord
Prostaglandin
Protein in Diet
Protein in Urine
Psychoprophylaxis
Pudendal Block
Puerperium

Q
Quickening

R
Recurrent Abortion
Registration of the Birth
Relationships
Relaxation
Respiratory Distress
    Syndrome
Responses of a Newborn
    Baby
Rest
Retained Placenta
Retroverted Uterus
Rhesus Disease
Rhesus Factor
Ripening of the Cervix
Rooming-In
Rubella

S
Savage, Wendy
Scan
Second Stage of Labour
Sex after the Birth
Sex in Pregnancy
Shared Care
Shave of Pubic Hair
Shirodkar Stitch

Show
Siblings
Sickle Cell Disease
Sickness
Signs of Labour
Signs of Pregnancy
Skin in Pregnancy
Sleep after the Birth
Sleep in Pregnancy
Small-for-Dates
Smear Test
Smoking
Sore Nipples
Special Care
Sphygmomanometer
Spina Bifida
Spotting
Squatting
Sticky Eye
Stillbirth
Stitches
Stress Incontinence
Stretch Marks
Sugar in Urine
Suitcase for Hospital
SVD
Swelling
Syntocinon

T
Tear in Perineum
Teeth in Pregnancy
Term
Thalassaemia
Third Stage of Labour
Threatened Miscarriage
Thrombosis
Thrush
Tiredness
TNS
Topping and Tailing
Toxaemia
Tranquillisers
Transition
Transverse Lie
Trial of Labour
Trilene
Trimester
Triplets

Trophoblast
Twins

U
Ultrasound
Umbilical Cord
Urinary Tract Infection
Urination
Urine Test
Uterus

V
V-BAC
Vacuum Extraction
Vagina
Vaginal Discharge
Varicose Veins
Venereal Disease
Ventouse
Vernix
Vitamin K
Vitamins
Vomiting in Labour
Vomiting in Pregnancy
Vulva
Vulval Haematoma

W
Washing Baby
Water Retention
Waters
Weighing Baby
Weight Gain of Baby
Weight Gain of Mother
Womb
Woolwich Shells
Work during Pregnancy

X
X-Rays

Y
Yellow Skin

Z
Zygote

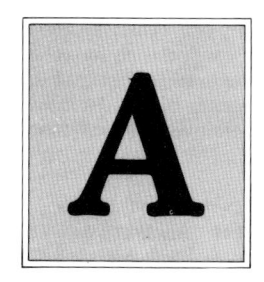

ABDOMEN Your tummy area. The word is used to describe the visible part of your body that enlarges during pregnancy, due to the growth of the womb or *uterus*. It also refers to the area inside the body: the uterus becomes an abdominal organ in pregnancy.

ABORTION Technically, an abortion happens when a pregnancy ends before 28 weeks. But in layperson's language, an abortion is a pregnancy that's deliberately ended. The other sort – 'spontaneous abortion' in doctorspeak – we call a *miscarriage*. In this country, abortion is legal, providing it's done by a doctor and follows the correct procedure. The earlier on in pregnancy an abortion is performed, the better – an early abortion is quicker, safer, and the indications are that it's easier to cope with emotionally. Late abortions are sometimes inevitable, however, for a variety of reasons. Currently, debate on the abortion issue centres around the upper age limit of the fetus. The legal limit is 28 weeks, beyond which the fetus is thought to be viable – that is, capable of life outside the mother. This is now untenable, say many people: fetuses much younger than 28 weeks have survived because of medical advances in the care of pre-term infants. In practice, few doctors agree to perform very late abortions; they point to the fact that there can be doubts about the age of a fetus, and that estimates of age can be wrong by as much as four weeks.

ACCELERATION OF LABOUR This describes the process undertaken when labour is already underway, but it's decided to speed it up for one reason or another. This can be done by *artificial rupture of the membranes* or by setting up an *oxytocin* drip, which puts a contraction-stimulating drug directly into the woman's bloodstream. This is done fairly commonly, but recent thinking suggests it's not invariably a good idea. Prolonged labour that isn't making sufficient progress can be tiring (and even dangerous) for both mother and baby, and of course no one wants a return to the time when women were in labour quite literally for days. However, labour does stop and start quite naturally in some women, and a change of position, or a spell of walking around, can start it off again. The disadvantage with drips in particular is that they can make the contractions too strong to cope with. This in itself can cause distress to the fetus, but it's even more likely that the mother will need more pain relief than she would otherwise have had. Rupturing the membranes is less 'interventionist' than a drip, and in many cases may be a better first option.

If you'd prefer to avoid acceleration – and don't forget, there are times when it's a good thing – and it's put to you during labour as a way of making you progress better, ask if you can move around or change position first, to see if that makes any difference.

ACTIVE BIRTH This is a way of giving birth that's grown in popularity in the last few years. It's more than just a 'method' – it's an approach that gives the mother and her partner responsibility for labour and birth, and a way of returning to a more instinctive, less rule-orientated behaviour. For instance, proponents of active birth favour allowing the woman to choose the position she wants for labour and delivery; if she's relaxed and in tune with her body's needs, she will tend to adopt the 'right' position that makes her feel best, and she will change from it when necessary. This, it's suggested, will make her labour more enjoyable and more comfortable, and will help her to make the most of her body's resources. It means that she may end up delivering on all-fours or perhaps in a squatting position – hardly ever on her back. This needs to be compared with the usual hospital procedure, which is to place a labouring woman propped up or on her back, from where she doesn't move until after her baby is born.

The approach is also diametrically opposed to most 'breathing' methods of *relaxation*, meant to relieve pain by various techniques specifically learnt and practised. Active birth gets beyond the conscious mind and urges women to seek out ways of experiencing birth on a deeper emotional level. Supporters also encourage women to question routine medical practices that could interfere with, and even sabotage, a normal physiological birth. Many midwives, and some doctors (notably Michel Odent in France) support active birth, or at least the individual's right to choose it as an option. There are a number of teachers of active birth, and the ideas are greatly influencing other ante-natal teachers (see *birth positions*, Useful Addresses and Booklist).

ACUPUNCTURE This is an ancient Oriental form of therapy, and there are a number of trained practitioners in this country. In brief it involves tapping life forces and energy, sometimes by the strategic and painless insertion of needles into defined points in the body. In childbirth, it's been used in this country, apparently with some success, as a form of pain relief. If you're interested in this aspect of it, you'd need to get your hospital's agreement, and you'd also need to find a properly qualified acupuncturist (see Useful Addresses).

ADOPTION These days, there are far fewer children available for adoption than there used to be. Those that are available tend to be older and they may also have physical, mental and/or emotional difficulties of varying degrees. Because there are so few children, adoption agencies (often run by the local authority) can be very selective in who they choose to be parents, and the very special needs of many of the children must justify this approach. It can lead to apparent unfairness, however, when prospective parents are 'rejected', told they're already 'too old' in their mid-30s. For information on adoption or fostering contact your local Social Services.

AFTERBIRTH Another word for the *placenta*, so-called because it is delivered after the birth of the baby, during the *third stage of labour*.

AFTERPAINS These are sensations – often quite strong – felt by new mothers in the first days after the birth. They are the result of the uterus contracting down to its non-pregnant state. Some women notice them particularly when they are breastfeeding, as the release of the hormone *oxytocin* caused by breastfeeding also stimulates contractions.

AGE OF MOTHER If we only ever considered the physical side of being pregnant and giving birth, we'd have to look at the statistics and say the best time for giving birth has to be in your early 20s to early 30s. This is the age where there's least likelihood of complications. Young girls still in their teens tend to have longer and more difficult labours, and so do older women in their late 30s and 40s. Older women have a greater possibility of giving birth to babies with *Down's syndrome* too. Having said that, however, the majority of babies born to women in all age groups are born healthily and happily after a normal labour!

Becoming pregnant is a social decision, too. And though it's probably not a good idea to start having babies in your teens (common sense tells you you've got a lot of living to do yet), it might be right for you as an individual, and not as a statistic. At the other end of the scale, it might not be until your 30s that your circumstances are right, in your view, for having a baby, and if you've had problems conceiving it might not be until late into your 30s or even after that you finally conceive. Each age has its problems and its advantages, and after all, you have to make up your mind for yourself. Remember, too, that parents themselves tell of the special joy and delight a 'late' baby brings to their early middle age!

AID Artificial Insemination by Donor. This is a treatment for infertility where the male half of a partnership has been diagnosed subfertile or infertile. The doctor places semen collected from a donor high up in the woman's vagina, through the cervix, and theoretically conception follows. The procedure has to be carried out as near as possible to the time of *ovulation*.

The whole issue of AID is clouded with moral, legal and clinical dilemmas. What is the legal status of an AID baby? Should he be denied the truth of his own conception? If the marriage breaks up, should the husband have a father's rights and obligations to the child? How can the couple be sure each one of them is equally happy about AID? And should doctors 'play God' and withhold AID from single women and lesbians?

Despite all these and many other questions, AID remains a popular form of treatment. It's available under the National Health Service in some areas. Semen donors are carefully screened for health or genetic defects and are matched as far as possible for physical characteristics to the male partner. Semen is stored in refrigerated sperm banks until required. One estimate is that 2000 AID babies are born each year.

AIH Artificial Insemination by Husband. This means the male partner's semen is used to inseminate the woman, but by placing the semen in the vagina manually, not by intercourse and ejaculation into the vagina. When it's carried out by a doctor he will usually place the semen through the cervix. It may be done when physical or emotional difficulties prevent actual penetration, but it's more often carried out to increase the chances of conception when the man's sperm count is low, or when sticky or 'hostile' mucus at the cervix prevents the sperm having an easy journey.

ALCOHOL Although a socially acceptable stimulant, the problem in pregnancy is that alcohol can be harmful to the fetus, and the present state of knowledge indicates that a safe amount of alcohol in pregnancy is unknown. There are various theories as to how exactly alcohol affects a growing baby, but it seems clear that even relatively small amounts can have an effect, and there's some evidence to show that this is particularly true if the fetus is at a crucial stage of development. Continuous heavy drinking can produce fetal alcohol syndrome, where the baby is born very *light-for-dates* with various physical and mental deficiencies. Over the years, expert advice to women has changed about what constitutes a safe upper limit of alcohol in pregnancy. The safest advice now is to stop drinking when planning a pregnancy or reduce your intake to no more than the occasional alcoholic drink. The alcohol concentration in your blood is the same as the alcohol level in your baby's blood, as alcohol crosses the placental barrier unchanged. Some women find cutting it out easier than others – they simply go right off the taste of alcohol in pregnancy.

ALLERGIES It's thought that a tendency to some allergies is inherited. If you or your family has a history of asthma or eczema, for instance, then your unborn baby is reckoned to stand a higher chance of suffering from similar symptoms. One way to protect him against this could possibly be to breastfeed exclusively, without even one bottle of formula milk, for at least the first three or four months, and delay the introduction of foodstuffs such as wheat and egg (common allergens) until the age of 8 or 9 months. This gives your baby time to mature and to develop his own allergy-protective mechanisms.

ALL-FOURS

There's no guarantee that following this advice will leave your baby allergy-free; and in fact recent research has thrown a great deal of doubt on it. One of the problems rests in the fact that not enough exclusively breastfed babies have been studied (that is babies who have had nothing but breast milk) to draw any firm conclusions. What isn't in doubt, however, is that some babies are allergic to cow's milk, including baby formulas based on it. When the mother isn't breastfeeding, the usual solution is to prescribe a baby formula based on soya instead.

ALL-FOURS A position preferred by some women for the *second stage of labour*, that is when the baby is actually delivered. It involves the mother kneeling, with her arms forward and straight, or leaning forward on her elbows, whichever feels most comfortable.

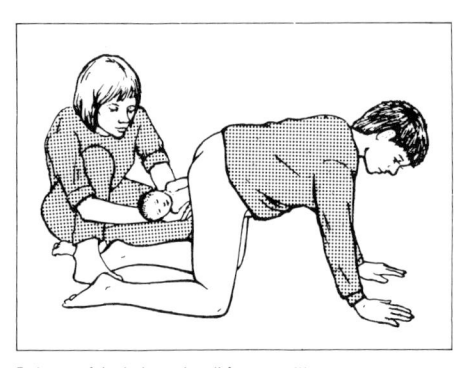

Delivery of the baby in the all-fours position.

It can be used during labour as well, and some women combine it with a rocking motion, which can be helpful and relaxing during a contraction (see *positions in second stage*).

ALPHAFETOPROTEIN (AFP) This is a substance in the *amniotic fluid*, and also present in the blood of pregnant women. If a blood test reveals AFP is in a high concentration, it can indicate the presence of a fetus with *anencephaly* or open *spina bifida*. There may be a raised level in women threatening to miscarry. However, it usually means nothing more than the mother is later on in pregnancy than she thought she was; is expecting twins; has a perfectly normal baby with a high AFP level. Many hospitals test the mother's blood for AFP at about 16 weeks of pregnancy. If there's a high level, she'll be asked to have further tests to check for the explanation. Some centres can carry out a spinal scan by ultrasound to get detailed information. The other accurate way of assessing the fetus is by *amniocentesis*.

The problem with routine AFP testing is that many mothers can be made anxious quite unnecessarily. Amniocentesis for instance, may be reassuring if it's negative, but this result won't be obtained until a few weeks have passed since the original blood test. Also amniocentesis itself is not without risks. Some authorities feel AFP testing should be offered only to women known to be at risk of bearing an affected child, mainly women who have already had one child with a neural tube defect.

AMENORRHOEA *(ay-men-or-rée-a)* The absence of menstrual periods. In a sexually active woman under the age of about 45, pregnancy is the most likely cause of amenorrhoea. After childbirth, you're unlikely to see the immediate return of your periods if you breastfeed. Some women find their periods return after a couple of months, others when their babies start taking foods other than breast milk. Others don't have a period until after they have stopped breastfeeding completely. Amenorrhoea can also occur after stopping the contraceptive pill – it's almost always temporarily.

AMNIOCENTESIS *(am-nee-o-sen-tée-sis)* This is a test which may be performed during your pregnancy. It may be done if there is considered to be a risk of your child suffering from certain handicaps. The test is done in hospital and it involves drawing off a sample of the *amniotic fluid* surrounding the baby. It's

4

AMNIOCENTESIS

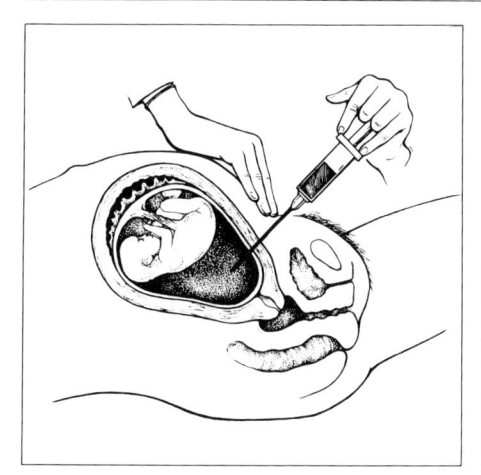

The position of the fetus is checked first by an ultrasound scan. The skin surface is numbed with local anaesthetic before a needle is inserted just above the pubic bone. Once the needle has reached the amniotic cavity, a sample of fluid can be withdrawn.

usual to have an *ultrasound* scan before the amniocentesis, so the doctor can assess where the baby is lying in the uterus. You don't usually need to stay in hospital, as amniocentesis is quite quickly and painlessly done (though mothers who have had it say they feel a sort of 'popping' sensation). The needle goes into the uterus through the abdomen which is first 'numbed' with local anaesthetic, and the fluid sample is drawn off into the syringe. The sample is then sent to the laboratory for testing and analysis. The wait for a result can be up to three weeks or so, as the tests involve growing a cell culture in the laboratory.

Chromosomal disorders – the most common one being *Down's syndrome* – can be detected, as can *neural tube defects*. Because the sex of the fetus can also be detected, amniocentesis is sometimes used when there's a risk of a sex-linked disorder (such as haemophilia, present only in males) being inherited from a parent. Amniocentesis in these cases is done when you are about 16 weeks pregnant.

In later pregnancy, a sample of amniotic fluid can be taken to assess the maturity of a baby's lungs. This can help an obstetrician decide whether to induce a fetus who isn't growing well (or to deliver by *caesarean section*). He needs to know whether the fetus is better off out the uterus rather than in and lung-functioning is an important aspect of this.

There is a risk with amniocentesis, particularly when it's done in the first half of pregnancy, that the test itself causes a miscarriage or *ante-partum haemorrhage*. This risk is reckoned by one medical expert to be in the region of 1.5 per cent. For this reason alone, it's not a test that's offered routinely. It's usually only done when there is a definite risk of handicap, for instance if the mother is in the older age bracket and therefore more at risk of Down's syndrome, or where raised AFP (*alphafetoprotein*) levels in her blood indicate the possibility of a neural tube defect. Another disadvantage is that the test can show a false positive, that is, the test may show the fetus to be handicapped, but in reality he is perfectly normal. And because the test shows up minor chromosomal disorders as well as the grosser ones, it raises the question of whether minor disorders should designate 'handicap' or not. All this means, of course, that you need to go into amniocentesis after some thought, and preferably after the chance to discuss all the implications at length with your doctor. You should realise that the main point of amniocentesis is to offer you a termination (abortion) if the fetus is handicapped, though of course you don't have to take up this offer. However, the major spin-off from an 'all-clear' amniocentesis could be peace of mind for the rest of your pregnancy, and that could be worth a lot to you. In the future, we may be able to look forward to a time when ultrasound techniques become sophisticated enough and sufficiently widely available to detect neural tube defects without the risks to normal babies of amniocentesis, though ultrasound itself has come under recent questioning. Work on *chorion villus sampling* means that certain defects may show up as early as eight weeks of pregnancy. An abortion as early as this is far

5

AMNIOTIC FLUID

less traumatic than one performed at 20 weeks or even later, which is the earliest possible date after a positive amniocentesis result. Other promising detection work is being done on *trophoblast* cells.

AMNIOTIC FLUID The amniotic fluid – also known as liquor – is pale in colour and it's contained in the *amniotic sac* forming the bag of waters. It's in this that the baby floats all the way through pregnancy. It cushions her from any knocks and jolts. The amount of fluid varies throughout pregnancy, decreasing slightly in the last few weeks. Samples of amniotic fluid can be taken during pregnancy in a process known as *amniocentesis* and then analysed. Because the fluid contains small amounts of skin tissue shed by the fetus, important genetic information can be detected on analysis. When there's an excess of amniotic fluid, the condition is known as *polyhydramnios*; an abnormally small amount is known as *oligohydramnios*. Both conditions can indicate certain problems – for example, *diabetes* in the mother with polyhydramnios.

AMNIOTIC SAC The bag of waters inside the uterus containing the *amniotic fluid*. It's formed of two thin membranes, and it's these membranes that rupture or break at the start of or during labour – and the result is that the amniotic fluid leaks out. In hospital, the membranes may be broken by the midwife in order to start labour off or to accelerate one that's already underway (see *artificial rupture of the membranes*).

ANAEMIA A lack of *haemoglobin* in the red blood cells. In pregnancy, the major cause of anaemia is a lack of *iron*, which is an important mineral normally taken in the course of a good, daily diet.

The effects of anaemia are mainly tiredness and lethargy, and in severe cases the efficiency of the placenta in getting oxygen to the fetus is affected. Your haemoglobin level will be checked during your pregnancy to see if you have any signs of anaemia.

ANAESTHETIST A doctor specialising in anaesthetics. If you had a general anaesthetic (with a *caesarean section* perhaps) the anaesthetist would give it. He would also perform an *epidural anaesthetic*.

ANALGESIA Pain-relief. An analgesic is a drug used to relieve *pain*. The commonest analgesics used in labour are Entonox (gas and air) and *Pethidine*.

ANENCEPHALY *(an-en-kéf-ally)* An invariably fatal defect of the central nervous system. The fetus doesn't develop a brain properly, and this leads to stillbirth or to death in the first few days after birth. Anencephaly is one of the *neural tube defects*.

ANKLES, SWOLLEN It's very common to have a slight degree of fluid retention in mid to late pregnancy, and round the ankles is a place where this fluid often gathers. It's not usually a cause for concern unless its onset is very sudden, if the degree is very severe or if it's seen in combination with other symptoms (for example high *blood pressure*). In these instances, it can be a sign of *pre-eclampsia*. Having a rest, with your feet up, can help reduce the swelling (see *oedema*).

ANTE-NATAL
Before birth.

ANTE-NATAL CARE Throughout pregnancy, most women have some form of ante-natal care. It can take a number of forms: all appointments can be at the hospital where you intend to have your baby, or you can have some appointments there and others with your GP and/or *community midwife*, or in some cases the community midwife might visit you at home for some appointments. (Women expecting a home confinement mightn't have any hospital appointments at all, unless the GP wanted a specialist opinion on some

ANTE-NATAL CLASSES

aspect of their pregnancy.) You might have a total of ten or eleven ante-natal checks, during your pregnancy.

The basic premise behind ante-natal care is that potential problems with pregnancy itself, or with labour and birth, or perhaps with the baby after the birth, can be spotted and perhaps averted, or at least lessened in severity. And good ante-natal care can make a real difference to a variety of situations: diabetic mothers, mothers having twins, mothers with high blood pressure, as well as mothers with non-medical problems – all may be helped with advice and treatment.

However it's not all good news. The way ante-natal care is handled in this country can be impersonal, dismissive of a woman's experience and feelings and anxieties; waits in clinics can be literally hours long; continuity of care – seeing the same staff at each appointment – seems impossible to arrange in most hospitals. There would seem to be a good case to be made out for carrying out at least some ante-natal checks in a mother's own home, with the community midwife visiting her. In any case, many women are discovering for themselves the relative ease in attending a local health centre clinic, instead of the hospital ante-natal clinic. Health centre clinics are run by GPs with community midwives; mothers report that the visits are much shorter, and the advantage of getting to know a smaller number of staff is that worries and anxieties can be more freely discussed. This is known as shared care. Even so, almost all women will need to visit the hospital ante-natal clinic at some time, and women with *high-risk* pregnancies will need to because this is where the consultant obstetricians are based.

Ante-natal care can only go so far in improving the health of pregnant women and their babies. The general health of a mother, her housing conditions, diet, education, lifestyle, her previous medical history – all things that prevail before she comes within a hundred miles of an ante-natal clinic – have a great impact on her chances of producing a healthy child after a problem-free pregnancy. Of course we do need ante-natal care, to sort out the high-risk sheep from the low-risk goats (without making us feel we're in a cattle market!), so that resources can be directed to those of us who need them most. But education and a better level of health for everyone will play their role, too, in the years leading up to parenthood.

ANTE-NATAL CLASSES Six, seven or eight classes (usually) held to prepare you for birth and parenthood. They normally contain information on keeping healthy during pregnancy, too. Fathers are sometimes invited, either throughout, or for one or two classes, and some courses are designed with couples in mind. The two main sources of ante-natal teaching in this country are via the National Health Service (the classes are held in a room in the hospital where you are to have your baby, or at your local health centre) and the National Childbirth Trust, a nationwide charity with the slogan 'education for parenthood'. There's no official, national syllabus for either NHS or NCT classes, and the style can vary according to who is taking the class.

The NHS classes are usually taken by a *midwife* and/or physiotherapist in the hospital, and *community midwife* and/or *health visitor* in the health centre. A doctor at the hospital may chip in with a talk on pain relief and perhaps caesarean sections. There's usually a film for one class, too. There'll be breathing and relaxation exercises and often a talk on breast and bottle feeding. In hospital, you may get the chance to look round the labour and delivery wards. Both sorts of NHS classes are free.

NCT classes are usually smaller than NHS ones, and though they too will cover similar ground preparing you for labour, birth and beyond, there may be more emphasis on class discussion and participation. You'll be encouraged to get involved in the decisions affecting the progress and outcome of your pregnancy. NCT teachers may or may not be midwives, but whatever they are they are women who will have undergone a thorough and wide-ranging training in all aspects of

ANTE-NATAL CLINIC

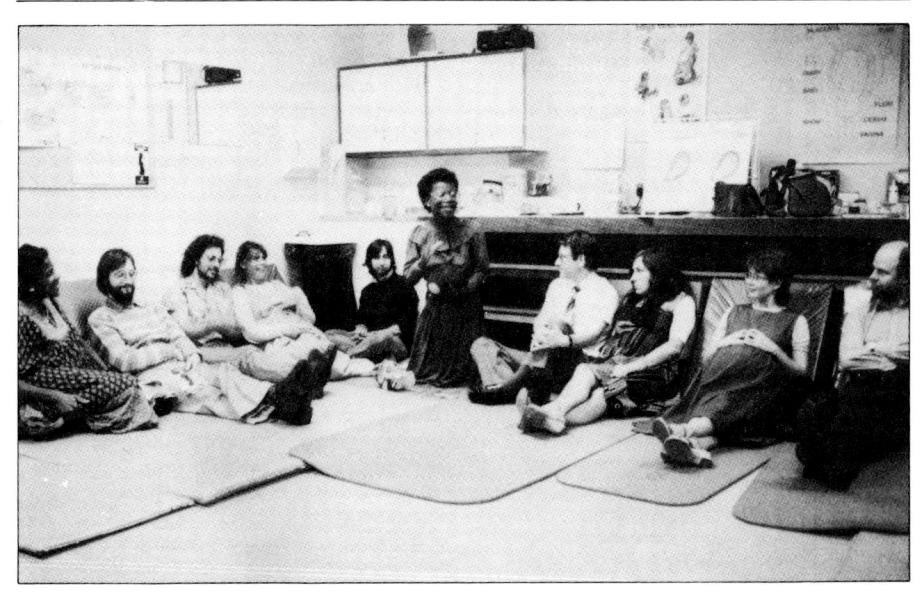

Many antenatal classes welcome fathers, too.

pregnancy, labour and parenthood; essentially they are well-informed and sympathetic laypeople, and often a useful counterpoint to the professionals you'll meet elsewhere in pregnancy. NCT classes aren't free and the charge varies from area to area.

Information on NHS classes can be had from your midwife; for NCT classes see your local branch. Local Birth Centres will know of other sorts of classes available in your area (see Useful Addresses).

ANTE-NATAL CLINIC This is where maternity unit staff – midwives and doctors – examine pregnant women. Your urine, blood pressure and weight will be checked at each visit, and you will have blood tests at some visits. The longest appointment (barring delays at others!) is your *booking appointment* which is usually the first visit. All specialist testing – *ultrasound* for example – takes place at the hospital, even if you are only visiting the clinic a few times, and getting the rest of your care from your GP.

If you have a choice of hospital, the waiting time and the organisation of their ante-natal clinic is something you can take into account; ask recently delivered women what their experience has been. The ideal clinic would be friendly, efficient, and held in a pleasant, welcoming part of the hospital, with facilities and toys for toddlers. Ideal clinics do exist – and I think their numbers are increasing (see *ante-natal care*).

ANTE-PARTUM HAEMORRHAGE A serious complication of pregnancy, and one which needs immediate medical attention. It's defined as bleeding from the site of the placenta after 28 weeks of pregnancy. When it's left untreated (unlikely of course with the right sort of attention), it's life-threatening to the mother as she can lose a lot of blood. It's obviously dangerous for the baby too, as it's caused by the placenta coming away from the uterus, and this directly affects the baby's nourishment. When the bleeding is severe or prolonged, the doctor might decide on a caesarean section in order to save the baby. If you start to bleed heavily in pregnancy, phone 999 for an ambulance and stress it's an obstetric emergency. However, many women these days at risk of APH are discovered in advance of any problems starting up. Such women may even be kept in hospital under observation (see *emergencies in pregnancy; placental abruption; placenta praevia*).

ANTERIOR LIP (OF CERVIX) Sometimes, at the very end of the *first stage of labour* when the cervix is all but fully dilated, the anterior or front lip of the cervix is still not completely taken up, as it must be to give a clear passage for the descent of the baby's head. This can mean that labour is rather slowed up, and though the mother may feel the urge to push, pushing is unproductive until that anterior lip is taken up with the rest of the cervix. The midwife can easily discover an anterior lip, because it can be felt as a small rim of cervix in front of the baby's head when she examines you. A few contractions later, and it's usually gone. You can help it on its way by kneeling down, with your head on the floor and your arms out in front of you. This position brings your baby forward a little bit, which helps the cervix retract, and it should also help you resist the urge to push.

ANTERIOR PRESENTATION The most usual presentation or position of the baby in the uterus. The front of his body is towards your backbone. It's also known as occipito anterior.

ANTIBODIES These are substances made by the body as a protective response to harmful diseases or foreign bodies. A rhesus negative mother carrying a rhesus positive baby may run the risk of producing antibodies to protect her own bloodstream against her baby's blood and bringing about *rhesus disease*. *Breast milk* supplies the baby with important antibodies to disease – something baby milk formula can't do.

ANTI-D GAMMA GLOBULIN This is given to a mother with rhesus negative blood to prevent her blood forming antibodies to her rhesus positive baby. The substance is usually injected after the birth of a rhesus positive baby to protect subsequent pregnancies (see *rhesus disease*).

ANXIETY IN LABOUR As during any life-changing event, labour can be an anxious time, particularly if you suspect for one reason or another that you could be in for a tricky delivery. Nevertheless, anxiety itself can interfere with the normal physiological processes of labour: the stress you feel can actually slow labour up and make it more painful. This is why so much ante-natal preparation concentrates on learning to relax. *Relaxation* not only helps us cope with the contractions of labour and delivery, it also helps to conserve and re-direct energy that's best used up on giving birth.

ANXIETY IN PREGNANCY A certain amount of anxiety is normal in pregnancy. Naturally, we worry about whether the baby's all right, and what sort of a world we are bringing a new baby into, whether we'll be okay as parents or not, and so on. But if your anxiety is preventing you from leading a normal life – keeping you awake, or creeping up on you and leaving you distressed and even panic-stricken – then seek advice. Drug-free treatment such as counselling or psychotherapy could help. Your GP can refer you for this.

APGAR TEST This is the standard test used to check the condition of a newborn baby, usually at one minute and five minutes after birth. The baby is given a score of 0, 1 or 2 for heart rate, muscle tone, breathing, skin colour and response to stimulation. Healthy babies in the best possible state after birth get 9 or even 10 out of a possible 10 points. Less than 7 after five minutes indicates there's some cause for concern, and under 4 means the baby is in severe difficulties and may require intensive care.

APNOEA MATTRESS *(ap-nee-a mattress)* This is a special mattress used with some sick or pre-term babies who are in danger of 'forgetting' to breathe. When breathing stops, the special alarms attached to the mattress are activated and a buzzer alerts staff (or parents if the baby's at home) to the situation. The baby is stimulated by touch or movement into breathing again.

APPEARANCE OF NEW BABY If your baby's healthy and born at term, he'll be pinkish in colour with soft, smooth skin. His hands and feet may be bluish at first. Black or brown babies are sometimes quite pale, and get darker over the first few days. Your baby may or may not have hair. He may be plumpish or skinny. If you have had a drug-free labour, he'll be alert and bright-eyed for the first hour or so after birth. Pre-term babies are quite scrawny to look at, and they are usually coated in *vernix*, which may also be on some full-term babies. Very pre-term babies have downy *lanugo* over their bodies. Late babies – *post mature* and born after 42 weeks – are sometimes thin, with dry, perhaps peeling or cracked skin (see *pre-term baby*).

ARTIFICIAL RUPTURE OF THE MEMBRANES Also known as amniotomy, it may be written in your notes as ARM. It's a procedure used to start labour off artificially (often combined with drugs to start the uterus contracting), or to accelerate a labour that's underway. The midwife punctures the amniotic sac enclosing the *amniotic fluid*, thus breaking your waters. The forewaters in front of the baby's head leak out through the vagina, and there is more room for the baby's head to descend. The hindwaters can also be broken. ARM makes the uterus contract more strongly than before.

The procedure doesn't usually hurt, if the membranes are ruptured after the cervix has started dilating. It's fairly routine in most hospitals. A lot of women's waters break quite naturally at the start of or during labour (though if the membranes are left alone many women will reach the end of the first stage with them still intact). However, ARM is being questioned – it could be, for instance, that the bag of forewaters acts as a cushion, protecting the baby's head during labour. You may prefer your waters to be left intact until they rupture naturally – let the midwife know. Nevertheless, if your labour is slow, and you don't mind a relatively non-invasive way of moving it along, ARM can help (see *acceleration of labour, induction*).

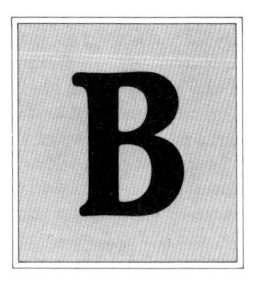

B

BABY CLINIC These are sometimes known as 'well' baby clinics because they are primarily there to monitor the development of healthy infants. If your baby is ill, you should take her to the family doctor. Your *health visitor* will tell you about your local clinic, when its sessions are and the sort of help and advice available from it. There's normally a routine weighing and the health visitor will also look at your baby and have a chat about any problems you may have. There may be a doctor in attendance at the clinic and your health visitor can refer your baby for an on-the-spot opinion if she thinks it's needed. The clinic is often where routine immunisation and developmental checks are done (see *weight gain of baby*).

BABY CLINIC

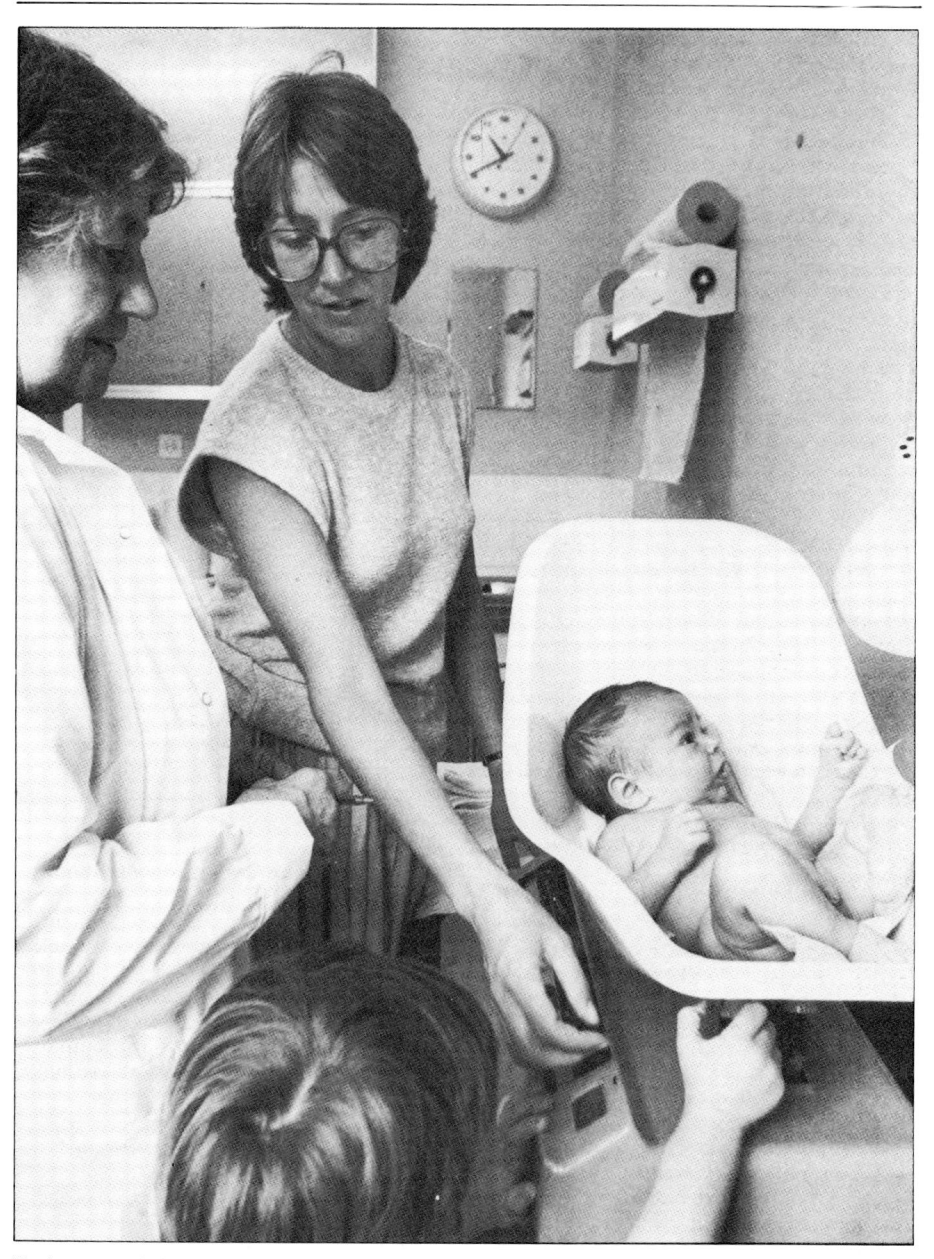

Weighing a young baby gives a guide to his general progress, when taken with other factors.

BACKACHE

BACKACHE This is not uncommon in pregnancy, and always worth reporting to your doctor, because it can very occasionally be a symptom of kidney infection. It's more likely to be caused by the general softening of ligaments in pregnancy and by your changing shape affecting your posture. To try and avoid backaches be sure to bend at the knees when picking something up, avoid carrying heavy loads, including shopping, for long distances, and wear comfortable low heeled shoes. Gentle all-round exercise like swimming can help, too.

Some mothers have a 'backache labour', when all the contractions are felt in the back. This can be the case when the baby is facing the 'wrong' way, that is, in a posterior position. Rubbing or massage by your labour companion can help.

BATH IN LABOUR Having a bath in labour is one of the usual procedures involved in *'prepping'* when you come into hospital – probably a hangover from the days when everyone who came into hospital was thought to be riddled with disease until proved otherwise. Nevertheless, having a bath can be a very soothing, even sensual experience in labour (though a standard hospital bathroom isn't very sensual, it has to be said). If you've had an enema, you may feel you actually need a bath to make you feel quite clean once more. Ask if your partner can be in the bathroom with you, if you would like this.

A hot bath is said to bring on labour (when you're ready anyway), so it's one thing to try if you're overdue and sick of waiting. There are occasional reports of mothers giving birth in the bath. In many cases, the mother just happens to be there because it's the most soothing place for her, rather than that she has chosen to have a 'water birth'. The babies come to no harm, of course, because they don't need to take in air through their lungs until after the umbilical cord is cut or has stopped pulsating. And after all, they've been in a bag of water all the way through pregnancy.

After delivery, a warm bath can be very refreshing, though in hospital you'll be given a good wash down straight after birth, and the chance to have a bath a few hours later.

BATHING BABY You'll probably be shown by your midwife how to bath your baby, but there aren't any really hard-and-fast rules about it, apart from the ones to do with safety. The main thing is to be sure your new baby doesn't get chilled, so ensure that the room is warm. Make certain the water is warm and not scalding (add warm/hot water after you've put the cold in to be sure you don't make any mistakes). Check the temperature with your elbow. It should feel pleasantly warm. Choose a mild soap or a baby bath additive, and soft towels, and have all his gear (clean nappy and clothes and so on) nearby so you don't have to go searching for bits you've forgotten. Baby baths can be useful, but a tiny baby will fit in a washing up bowl (though do buy a separate one for him!) and then he can move into the big bath – though as you have to hold him all the time this can be back-breaking for you.

You don't have to bath your baby every day. On days when you don't bath him, *'topping and tailing'* will do. Also you don't need to make bathtime a special time-by-the-clock; do what suits you best though avoid times when he is obviously hungry or tired.

Safety note: never ever leave a baby alone in the bath for even a moment. This includes babies old enough to sit up. Drowning accidents happen with tragic regularity.

BEARING DOWN This is what you do when your baby is about to be born. It's as if all your strength and energy resources are directed towards the birth of your baby. The sensation comes to most (though not all) women quite spontaneously after the cervix is fully dilated. Bearing down is rather like a massive urge to open your birth canal wide and push your baby out; there may be a feeling rather like the need to open your bowels, too, especially as your baby's head may be pressing on your rectum.

The way most women give birth in this country is by responding to encouragement to

BATHING BABY

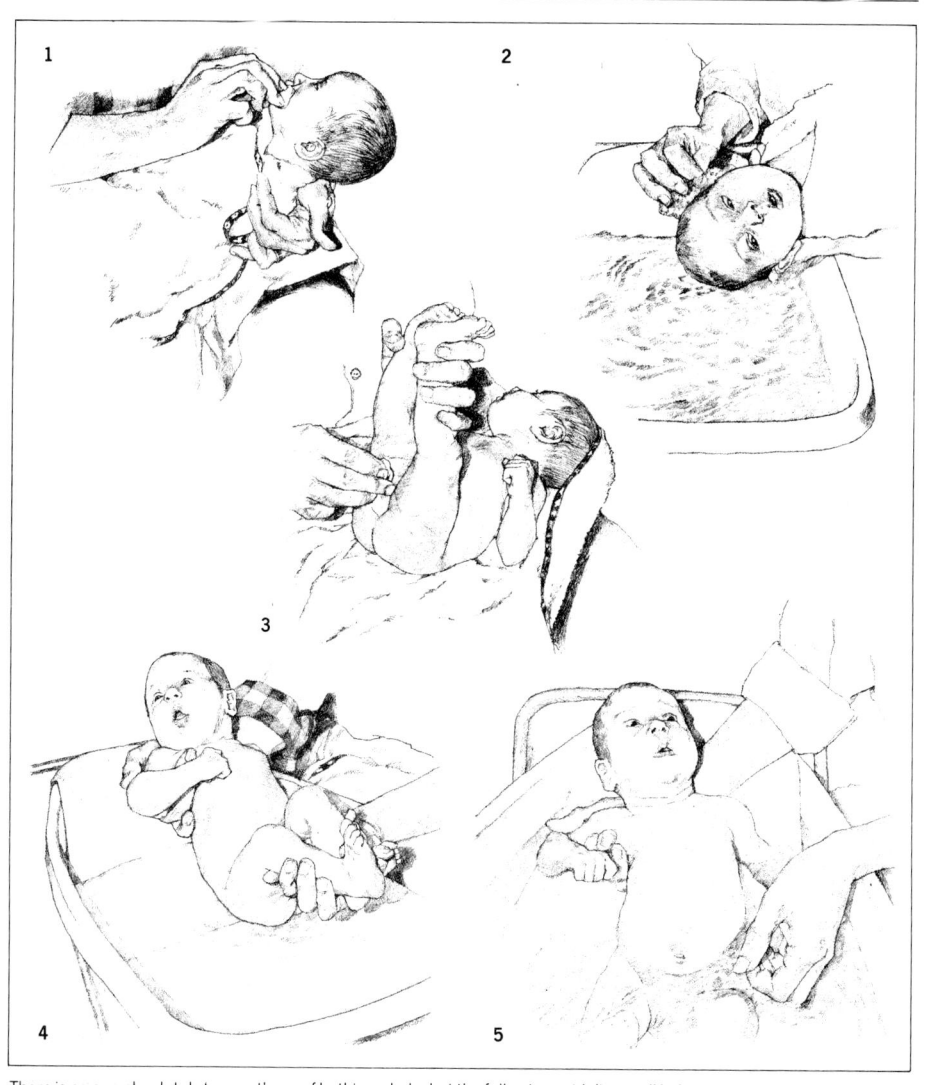

There is no one absolutely 'correct' way of bathing a baby but the following guidelines will help you.
1 Undress your baby apart from her nappy and wrap her in a towel. Wash her face and neck first with plain water and cottonwool or a soft face-cloth. Dry carefully.
2 Keeping your baby wrapped in the towel, lower her head over the side of the bath and soap and rinse her scalp.
3 Take off the nappy and wash your baby's bottom with soap and water.
4 Holding your baby under the shoulders and legs, as shown, lower her into the bath.
5 Continuing to firmly support your baby's shoulders, allow her to kick her legs and, using your free hand, soap and rinse her body.
Make sure you dry your baby gently and thoroughly after her bath.

give greater and more intense pushes. During the contractions of the second stage the midwife may tell you to push really hard, perhaps three or four times per contraction, holding your breath as you do so. This is being questioned, now, however. It could be that it's better to push according to what your body tells you, and this might mean shorter, more gentle pushes during some contractions, and longer ones during other contractions. Holding your breath as well as putting all that tremendous effort into pushing could certainly affect your baby adversely, too: you reduce the amount of oxygen your body is getting when you hold your breath, which slows down your blood flow and the blood supply to your baby can be affected by this, too. None of this will affect a healthy, strong baby for more than a few seconds, but it must make sense to study how the baby reacts, and to make sure we give him the best possible environment during his birth.

Bearing down can be done in many different positions, but growing numbers of midwives and doctors are giving women the chance to opt for an upright delivery, where it would seem that among other advantages, the bearing down contractions can be most effective (see *second stage of labour*).

BEDDING FOR BABY A baby doesn't need a pillow (in fact they're dangerous) until he's at least a year old. He'll need several sheets for cot/crib and pram (though you can use the same ones and fold to fit), and when you remember that even the best-pinned nappy doesn't always contain everything, and that babies can be sick several times a day, you'll be wise to stock up with at least seven or eight sheets. Old, soft and oft-washed bedsheets cut down make very good baby sheets, though the newer fitted stretchy sort have the big advantage of staying put over the mattress.

You'll also need at least two blankets for both cot and pram, and one or two more won't come amiss. The easiest-to-wash sort are cotton cellular blankets (the type used in hospitals) and they give warmth without bulk. They aren't, however, as pretty to look at as the other less basic sort. Some people buy duvets for their newborns, but I would probably err on the side of caution and avoid them for a tiny baby, rather than worry about suffocation. A plastic-covered mattress will probably come with the cot and the pram, but if your baby turns out to be very dribbly or sickly, or very leaky at the other end, you could buy a fitted waterproof sheet; this can be washed, to get rid of any smells that can linger even with plastic.

BEDREST This means staying in or near your bed for most of the day as well as all night. It's often recommended to women who threaten to miscarry, and in later pregnancy to women who have suffered some bleeding, or who have high blood pressure. Some women are admitted to hospital where the bedrest can be more likely to succeed as there's no distracting domestic routine or responsibilities. The condition needing the bedrest can be monitored more closely in hospital, too.

BICORNUATE UTERUS This is a rare malformation of the uterus. There is a complete or partial division down the centre of the uterus – almost as if there are two wombs. In even rarer instances there may be two cervixes and two vaginas. The condition can cause problems and miscarriage is one of them. Normal pregnancy and labour are sometimes possible, though, except the baby may lie in a less-than-ideal position because of the lack of space.

BIRTH Giving birth is something most women in this country do perhaps once or twice or thrice in their lives. This century has seen a great rise in the general level of our health, as well as a wide-ranging development in ante-natal care, and life-saving techniques applied during and after birth itself. The result is that going into labour and delivering is overwhelmingly likely to result in the birth of a live, healthy infant. The combination of

BIRTH

these factors – small families, safe childbirth – has meant that a mother's emotional investment in each birth is that much greater. We not only expect a hazard-free delivery and a perfect baby, we want the experience to be a happy and fulfilling one as well. And I think most women would feel we are right to want this. But because we are all different as individuals, our definition of a happy and fulfilling experience will differ too. For some it will mean the more-or-less guaranteed absence of pain, and they will opt for an *epidural*. Some women find the presence of high-tech *fetal monitors* and so on is very reassuring. Other mothers want to give birth as naturally as possible without drugs or medical intervention. And yet others feel the only way they can have the birth they want is at home. Risk-factors apart, the mood is becoming a feeling that the choice should be ours, after talking in partnership, not conflict, with the medical people involved (see *home birth; labour; pain in labour*).

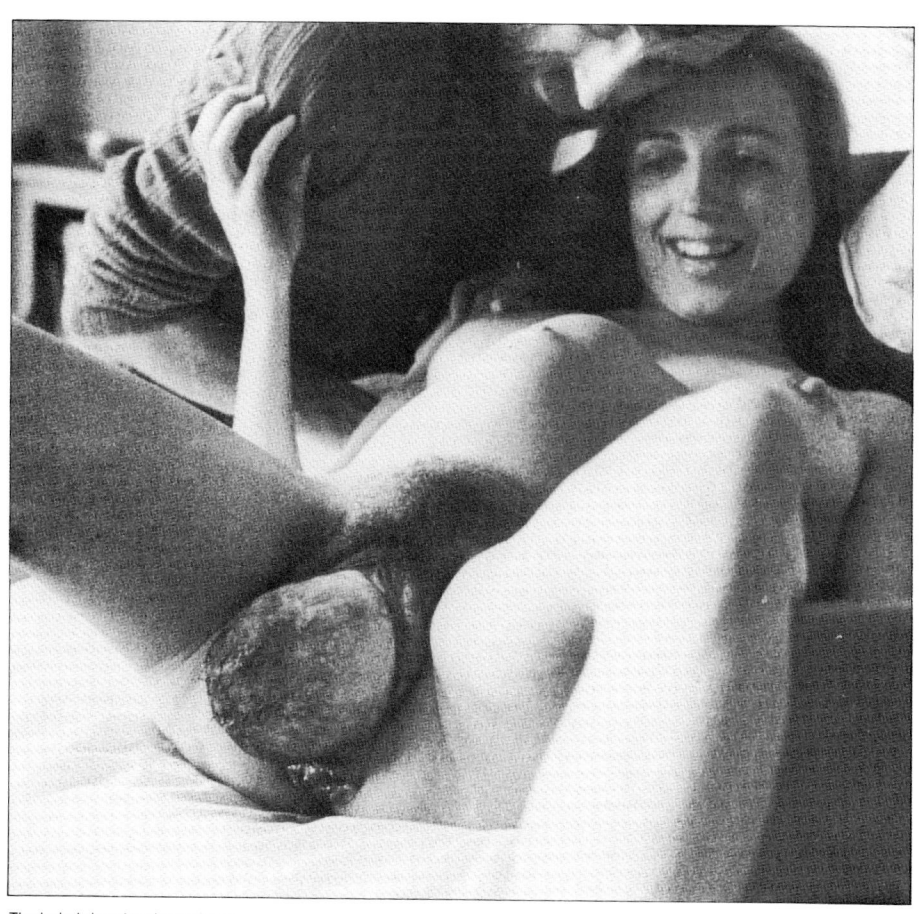

The baby's head is almost born.

BIRTH CERTIFICATE

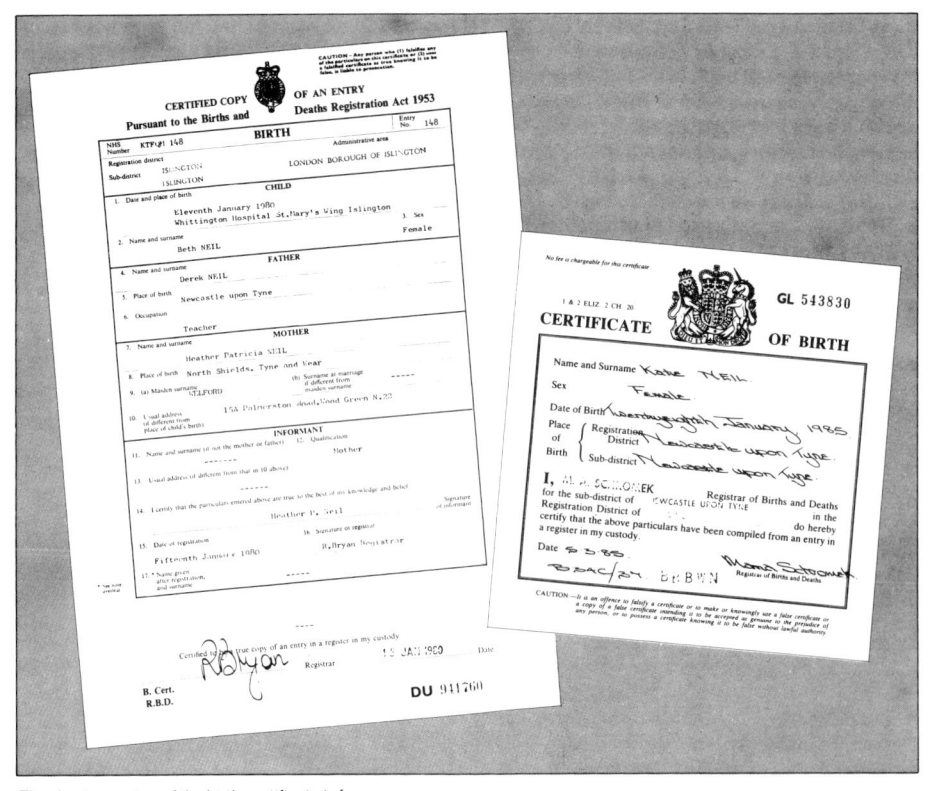

The shorter version of the birth certificate is free.

BIRTH CERTIFICATE Everyone has one and in fact, in this country, it's illegal to leave the birth of a baby unregistered. You have six weeks (three in Scotland) to register your baby's birth. If you aren't married, the baby's mother has to register the birth (if the baby's parents are married to each other, either one can register it) and the father's name can be included on the certificate only if he gives his consent, or if the court has awarded the mother an affiliation order stating the name of the father. As a result of all this, you have a birth certificate, in one or both of two versions, short and long – the long one contains more details (see *registration of the birth*).

BIRTH CHAIR An interesting 'new' idea in childbirth that in reality goes back many hundreds of years, and maybe even beyond that. There are Biblical references to birth chairs and stools, and it appears that many cultures and times have had a specially designed chair for giving birth in. These days, they're being looked at again, and the reports of women who have used them indicate that they could well offer a useful option to the various positions you can adopt during labour and birth.

Some hospitals have invested in expensive adjustable birth chairs, all chrome and leather-look upholstery, but plain chairs seem just as effective. The idea is to allow a

BIRTH POSITION

comfortable, upright position for the last part of labour and delivery. Some women have given birth on an upturned bucket, their upper bodies supported by their partner or birth attendant (see *positions for first stage; birth position*).

BIRTHING ROOMS A description of rooms designed for mothers to give birth in, but without the usual obvious presence of equipment, tiled walls and bare floors. A birthing room could look like a cosy bedroom in a normal family house, with the addition of large cushions, possibly a birth chair or stool, and/or a special birthing bed, and soft adjustable lighting (see *delivery room*).

BIRTHMARKS Lots of newborns have a few marks on them – pressure marks perhaps from *forceps*, or so-called stork's beak marks present most commonly on the forehead, neck or hairline. In the vast majority of cases, these marks disappear. Other marks may appear later – up to a few weeks after the birth – and the most common of these are strawberry marks, which are red and raised. These fade as well, though it can take a few years. Port-wine stains are flat and dark red, and these are permanent. Recent work with lasers has shown that there is hope for successful treatment for port-wine stains as well.

BIRTH POSITION One of the major aspects of the 'childbirth debate' that's filled newspapers and TV programmes over the last few years has been the position the mother is in when her baby is born. In many hospitals, a mother is put on her back, with her legs supported, either in stirrups, or supported by a medical attendant at each side. The big advantage of this is that the perineum and the

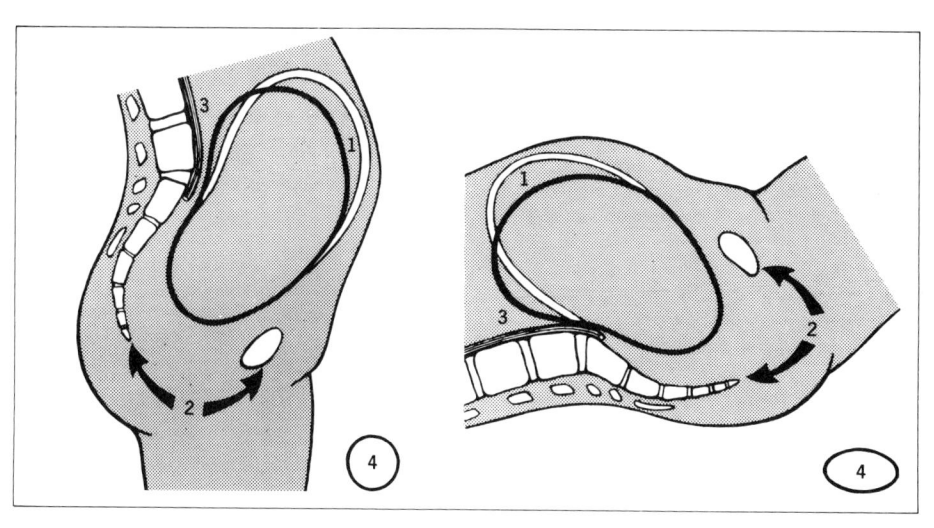

Advantages of being upright during labour and delivery.
1 Uterus contracts upwards and outwards.
2 Sacrum is 'freed' and space between sacrum and the pubic bone is enlarged.
3 Avoids compression of major blood vessels that might give rise to fetal distress.
4 Vaginal opening isn't compressed.

Disadvantages of lying on your back during labour and delivery.
1 Uterine contractions are acting against gravity and a natural inclination.
2 Space between sacrum and pubic bone reduced.
3 Major blood vessels compressed.
4 Vaginal opening compressed.

BIRTH POSITION

baby's head can be watched carefully (which is why the position is used with forceps) and midwives are trained to assess the progress of labour and the second stage from this angle – though not this angle alone, of course.

The disadvantages of the position are well-documented, and research has shown that keeping a mother lying down during the second stage (or during the first stage too) significantly reduces the blood supply to the uterus and the placenta, because the major abdominal vessels are compressed, as is the major artery of the heart, and this can adversely affect the baby, and make contractions more painful. The pelvic opening is at its widest in an upright position, and you can actually make it smaller if you lie down. Another disadvantage is that it's almost impossible for a mother to see her baby being born, and there's also some evidence to suggest that an episiotomy is more likely in this position.

Left to themselves, as they are in various other cultures, women tend not to adopt a lying-down position. They may change position a few times during the contractions of the second stage. Squatting, kneeling, all-fours, sitting, supported squatting (where another person holds you under your arms when you squat) – all are alternatives.

Whether you give birth at home or in hospital, it's a good idea to make sure you

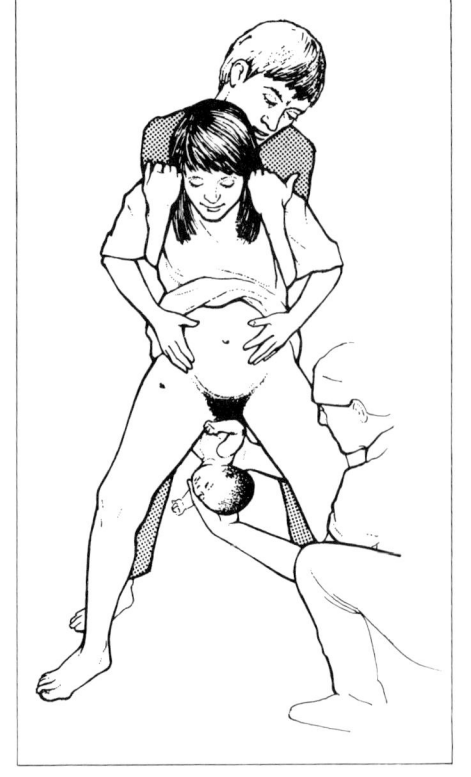

Standing supported squat

have plenty of pillows, and a chair or a stool in the room, so you can change your position at will. If you want to be free to choose your position when you give birth, ask at your ante-natal clinic what the current policy is. If there is a standard way of delivery, ask if you can have it included in your notes that if all goes well you wish to be able to choose. Practise different positions during pregnancy, and ask about them at ante-natal classes (see *birth chair; lithotomy position; positions for first stage*).

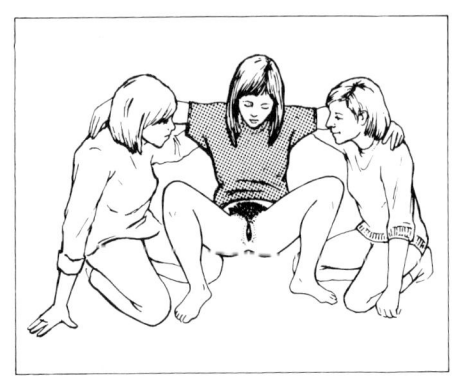

Sitting supported squat

18

BLOOD PRESSURE

BLADDER Where your urine is stored in the body. During labour it's a good idea to make sure you pass water regularly as the sensations of a contracting uterus may disguise the feelings of a full bladder, and a full bladder may hold up the progress of your labour.

BLASTOCYST The very early 'product of conception'. Once the egg has been fertilised by a sperm, it travels down the fallopian tube towards the uterus. As it does so, the single cell divides and multiplies and becomes what is called a blastocyst, which implants itself in the prepared lining of the uterus. The blastocyst is formed of two layers – the outer one eventually becomes the placenta, and the inner one becomes the fetus.

BLEEDING Any bleeding in pregnancy is potentially serious, and it should be reported to a doctor. Very light bleeding in early pregnancy is not uncommon, and often the pregnancy continues to progress without any further mishap. In later pregnancy, it can mean the placenta is starting to detach from the uterus, which of course is hazardous for the baby and it is important to seek the advice of your doctor immediately. It's important to remember that any blood loss in pregnancy comes from the mother's blood supply, and not the baby's, which could be reassuring if you have bled, and now find it's stopped.

It's normal to lose a certain amount of blood (up to about a pint) during labour and birth, and for between 2 and 6 weeks after, you will have a blood-stained discharge in gradually decreasing amounts, as the uterus sheds its pregnancy lining (the *lochia*). Any sudden or large loss of blood, though, could indicate something more serious and you should contact a doctor (see *ante-partum haemorrhage*).

BLIGHTED OVUM One of the many possible causes of *miscarriage*. It happens when the pregnancy fails to develop properly in the first few weeks, and though the woman's body may appear to have all the symptoms of pregnancy, such as lack of periods, a fetus never really starts developing. The result is always a miscarriage, usually in the first ten weeks. One authority suggests blighted ovum is due to an egg being fertilised by an abnormal sperm, but there's no way of preventing this in future pregnancies other than by trying to make sure both partners are as healthy as possible when they next wish to conceive.

BLOCKED DUCTS A complication of breastfeeding. If you suffer from *engorgement* or if your baby goes rather a long time between feeds (or has a bottle instead of a breastfeed), or if you are trying to keep her to a feeding routine, or sometimes if you're just unlucky, you can get a blockage of milk in one or more of the ducts leading to the nipple. The symptoms are a red patch of skin on the breast, together with a lump inside the breast. The breast may be painful to touch. It's important to get rid of the blocked duct or you could get an infection. A midwife, health visitor or breastfeeding counsellor will explain that you need to feed the baby to get rid of the blockage, and while feeding, to massage the lump towards the nipple. If it doesn't disappear within a day of this treatment, then you should see your doctor who may prescribe antibiotics to prevent any infection. It's important, whatever you do, not to stop feeding from the affected breast as this will make the problem worse. (*Expressing* your milk from it will also help to unblock the duct.) Avoid wearing *bras* that are too tight, or ones with a band across the top of the breast, as these can both cause a blockage. And don't get into the habit of pressing on your breast with your fingers while you feed, as this can also result in a blocked duct.

BLOOD PRESSURE This is the force or pressure of the blood on the walls of the blood vessels. It's measured by an instrument called a sphygmomanometer, which takes two readings: one records systolic pressure (the

19

BLOOD TESTS

maximum pressure when the heart is pumping); the other, the diastolic pressure (the pressure when the heart is at rest). The two readings are written into your notes one on top of the other (systolic on top, diastolic below) as in a fraction, for example, 130/80. The midwife will take your blood pressure at every ante-natal visit – it's a simple and absolutely painless procedure. You'll need to roll up your sleeve, so don't wear something that's too tight at the wrist.

If your blood pressure is unduly raised, or consistently high over a number of visits, it can be cause for concern. A raised blood pressure (or hypertension) can be a first sign of *pre-eclampsia*. Severe hypertension can also affect the health of the fetus. Blood pressure can rise as a reaction to stress, or tension. Waiting for a long time in an ante-natal clinic with a fractious toddler can be quite enough to give a temporary high reading. If this happens to you, many ante-natal clinics are happy to wait for ten minutes or so, while you consciously relax, and then the reading will be taken again. Consistently high blood pressure may mean you're advised to rest more during your pregnancy and in more severe cases, you may even be asked to come into hospital for *bedrest*. In some cases, drugs can control the hypertension.

Raised blood pressure is relatively common in first pregnancies (between 5 and 10 per cent are affected), and relatively unlikely to occur again in subsequent ones.

BLOOD TESTS During pregnancy you'll be asked to undergo a number of blood tests, and they are normally routine ones, taken to rule out serious disorders or to check everything is as it should be with your health. The list of what the hospital checks for varies from place to place, and if you've got a medical history that demands it, or if it's known you've already got a problem detectable by a blood test, you'll be asked to have further tests. Basically, however, a sample of your blood will be taken at your first ante-natal visit, and it will be sent to the laboratory to check for (1) *rubella* antibodies, to make sure you're immune to rubella; (2) *anaemia*; (3) your blood group, and whether you're rhesus positive or negative, to check for the possibility of *rhesus disease*; (4) *venereal disease*; (5) *sickle cell disease* if you are West Indian or West African. Your *haemoglobin* (Hb) level will also be checked from a further one or two blood samples taken later in pregnancy, and this helps diagnose anaemia if it should occur.

In many hospitals women are screened, via a blood test, for *alphafetoprotein* and this test can help diagnose *spina bifida* or *anencephaly*. In late pregnancy, some hospitals test for *oestriol* and/or human placental lactogen, two hormones which reflect the functioning of the placenta. They're routine tests in some units, whereas in others they're only done if there's some reason to suspect the baby isn't growing well enough.

Whenever your blood is taken for testing (a simple procedure, by the way, usually involving a fine needle being inserted into a vein in your arm – virtually painless), you should feel free to ask what is being looked at, though some clinics will volunteer this information. You should also be told the results of these tests; just a few words like 'Your blood tests show that everything's fine' can put a lot of women's minds at rest. If you're not told the results, do ask your doctor on your next visit.

BLOOD TRANSFUSION The process whereby a patient's blood is replaced or partially replaced by blood from a donor. In a mother, severe *ante-partum haemorrhage* or *post-partum haemorrhage* may mean she needs a blood transfusion, and in a new baby, a blood transfusion is very occasionally needed, for example in a baby with severe *rhesus disease* or in a pre-term baby who is badly anaemic.

BLOOM OF PREGNANCY Rather undefinable, but when you see it or when you've got it, you recognise it. Lots of women have a time in pregnancy – usually in the middle months – when they feel wonderfully healthy, and this shows itself in clear skin and hair and general vitality.

BLOOM OF PREGNANCY

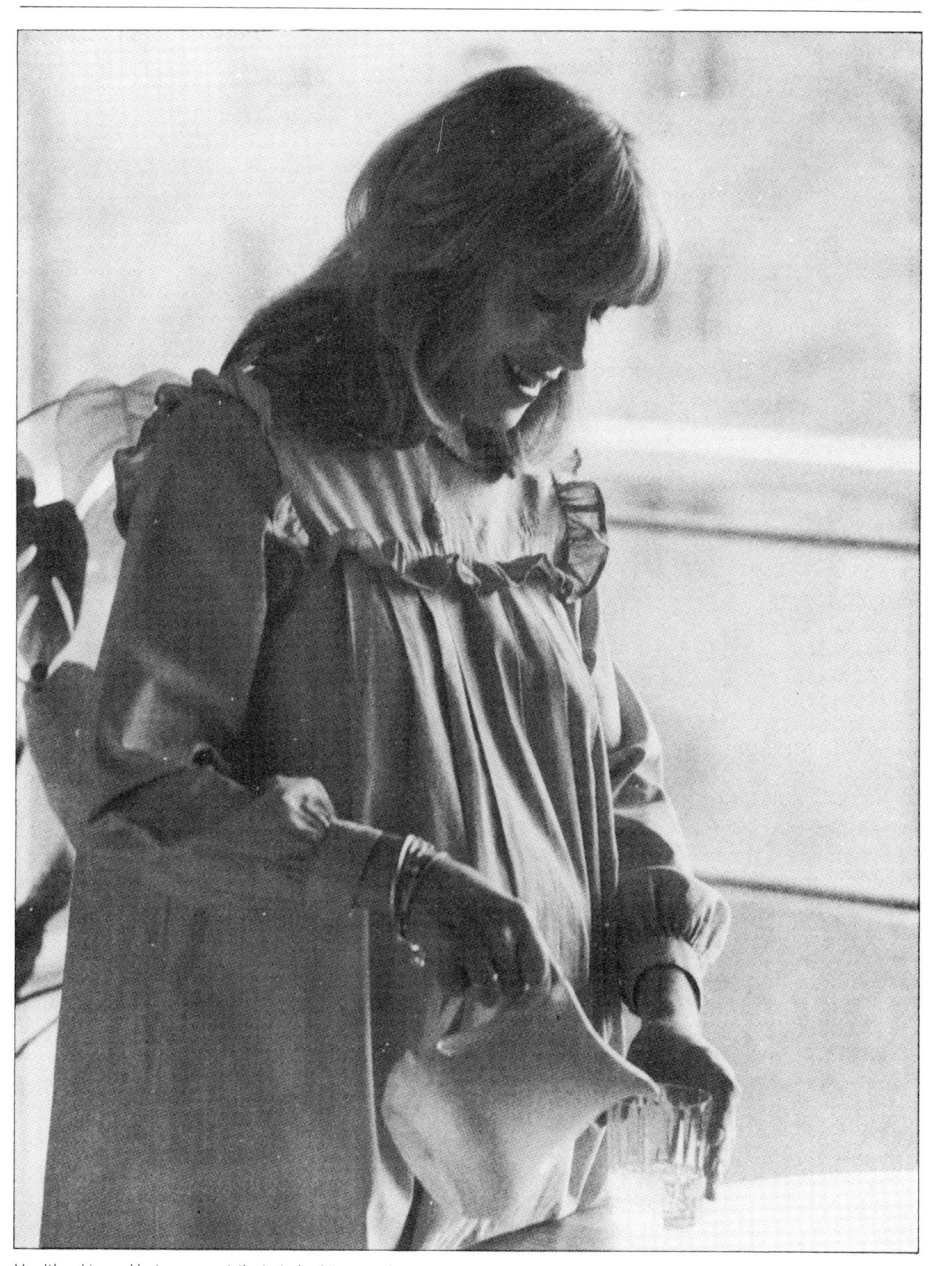

Healthy skin and hair can contribute to looking good in pregnancy, especially during the second three months.

BONDING

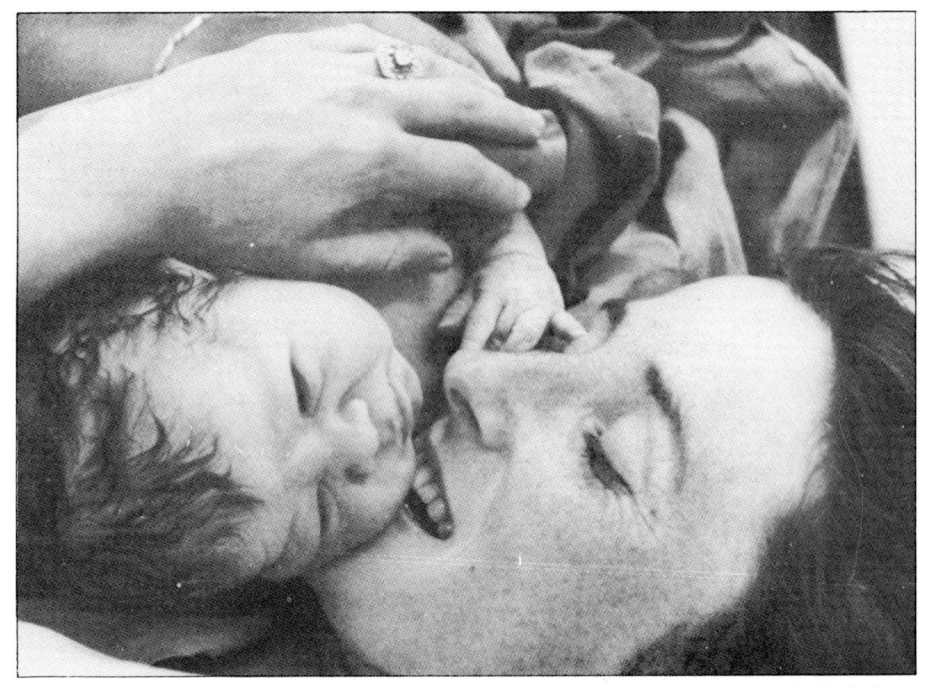

Close physical contact between mother and baby is important in the bonding process especially immediately after birth.

BONDING A rather over-worked word used to describe the process of attachment between a newborn and his parents. Two American researchers found that mothers given time soon after birth to see, touch and cuddle their new babies are less likely to have emotional and relationship problems with them later on. They say we need the chance to bond with our children in order to forge the social-biological link of love between us. The result of this research is that many more hospitals now allow a mother and father time alone with their child soon or even immediately after birth, which is very valuable and enjoyable for them.

Basically bonding is the establishment of a loving relationship between a parent and a child, but if circumstances dictate, it doesn't have to start straight after birth. Some mothers and babies are separated because of illness, and the process of getting to know and love the baby may take place while the baby is perhaps in *special care*. Many women find, in any case, that they take time to feel the strong maternal surge of feeling that others experience straight away; they gradually, rather than immediately, fall in love with their babies. This is normal, and it's just a variation of human behaviour.

BOOKING APPOINTMENT The first appointment at your ante-natal clinic, where you are formally accepted as a patient. It's usually the longest appointment as the midwife or doctor will ask a lot of information about you and your partner.

You will be asked the usual personal details – your age, date of birth, religion, the type of work you do, where you live – and similar questions will be asked about your partner. The midwife or doctor will also want to know about any illnesses or conditions in your, and your partner's, family (in case they can be passed on), and about your medical history – whether you have had any serious illnesses or operations. You may also be asked about what contraception you used before getting pregnant and about the pattern of your periods, in particular the date of the first day of your last period (this enables the midwife to work out your approximate delivery date). If you have been pregnant before details of this pregnancy will be recorded also.

Although it might seem rather early, the midwife or doctor may discuss your intentions regarding breast or bottle feeding. Take the chance to talk your ideas through.

You're usually asked to have *blood tests* done as well. Some hospitals like you to see a dietician and possibly the hospital social worker as well.

The booking appointment is a very good opportunity for you to discuss your pregnancy, labour and birth, and to ask about anything that worries you and get as much information as possible. It is also a chance for the hospital staff to get to know you too.

BOTTLE FEEDING The 'other' way to feed new babies. Although breast milk is the ideal and perfectly balanced food and drink, the bottle can be given by someone other than the mother, and in certain circumstances this can be important. It also supplies food for the baby without being affected by drugs or medication the mother is taking, or her diet. It avoids feelings of embarrassment or awkwardness that (sadly in my view) prevent some women from breastfeeding.

When feeding by bottle, it's important that only a specially formulated baby milk or expressed breast milk is used, and that scrupulous attention is paid to sterilising all feeding equipment. A baby fed on formula milk doesn't get his mother's antibodies to infection through her breast milk, and he may possibly catch an infection that could reach him through an improperly sterilised bottle or teat or whatever. The other reason for sterilising is that milk traces may get bacteria in them (warm milk goes off very easily, so don't leave a warm bottle around on the off-chance the baby will want it later. For the same reason, avoid those little thermal bottle containers. They're only useful to keep a feed *cold* until you can heat it up.) Follow the instructions on the baby milk tin when making up feeds, and if the formula doesn't 'agree' with your baby's digestion, speak to your doctor or health visitor before changing brands (see *feeding*).

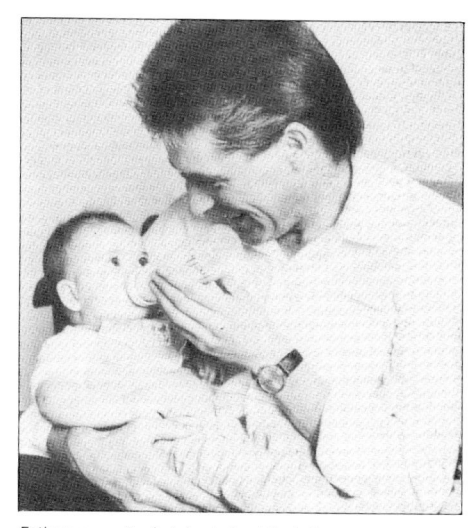

Fathers can enjoy helping to feed the baby, too.

BRAS Even if you don't normally wear a bra, you may well find you're more comfortable with one during pregnancy. Your breasts will enlarge, sometimes considerably, from the very beginning of pregnancy. If you really do have small breasts, and they remain on the small side, then you probably can get away without wearing a bra, though it could be that you run more of a risk of stretch marks if you don't wear one. You don't actually need a proper nursing bra until you're breastfeeding (and even then, many mothers just wear a normal bra) but it will save you having to buy them later on if you get them while you are pregnant. Whatever you get, make sure it's a good comfortable fit – it's worth getting it fitted professionally. If it's cotton, or cotton/polyester, it's likely to keep its shape with frequent washing better than nylon or stretchy material (you will need to wear a clean nursing bra at least once a day during the early weeks of breastfeeding). Choose a bra that offers good, firm support, has wide shoulder straps to stop them digging into your shoulders, and an adjustable fastening – not only do your breasts increase in size, but also your rib-cage as your pregnancy advances. When choosing a nursing bra avoid those with a drop cup and band of fabric across the top of the breast, which could lead to *blocked ducts*. If your breasts get very heavy, you may feel more comfortable if you wear a bra at night as well, and a sleep bra is a lightweight alternative if you don't think your breasts are in need of much support.

BRAXTON-HICKS CONTRACTIONS
These are 'practice' *contractions* of the uterus which you will probably only feel in the last weeks, though they occur all the way through your pregnancy. Unless you are very unlucky, the contractions aren't likely to be painful (and some women aren't aware of them at all). They are thought to be the uterus' way of preparing for the contractions of labour, though they differ in quality from true labour contractions by being irregular and short. You'll probably experience them as a sort of hardening and tightening across your tummy.

BREASTFEEDING Most women start off by breastfeeding their babies these days, though a proportion stop in the first days or weeks after birth. Motivation seems to be a strong factor: if you really want to breastfeed, you are likely to breastfeed for longer. Various aspects of breastfeeding are discussed elsewhere in this book, but perhaps the three most important points to remember are: (1) it's undoubtedly the best way to get your baby off to a healthy start in life – *breast milk* is nutritionally balanced, easily digested and helps to protect the baby from infections; (2) a good position on the nipple helps the baby suck efficiently and helps to avoid potential problems (see *latching on*); (3) feeding your baby on demand – whenever he's restless or appears hungry – is the best way to establish a good milk supply. If you need help with breastfeeding, ask your midwife, health visitor or doctor. Breastfeeding counsellors also offer help and advice, either in person or over the phone. They are specially trained volunteers and they are available any time you need them (see *feeding*, Useful Addresses).

BREAST MILK The best food for new babies, and the wonderful thing is we all produce it, even if we don't intend to feed our babies. It contains exactly the right balance of nutrients to suit a baby's digestion, and the composition of it actually changes as the baby grows. Mothers of pre-term babies make a milk that's higher in fats and other constituents – and giving your pre-term baby your own milk can be a very positive way of making your own unique contribution to his care. Breast milk also contains antibodies which help the baby build up resistance to infection.

Although everyone starts off with the ability to make breast milk, simply by virtue of having given birth (the delivery of the placenta sets off the hormonal reaction that triggers milk production), the supply of breast milk only continues if the baby sucks, or if the milk supply is stimulated by expressing milk. Interestingly enough, stimulation by a baby seems to be a minimum qualification for being able to produce breast milk, as mothers of adoptive babies have produced breast milk by suckling their babies frequently. This needs time, dedication, motivation and support, and almost always the baby needs additional feeds of formula milk. Adoptive mothers are more likely to succeed if they have been pregnant at some time in the past (see *colostrum*).

BREASTFEEDING

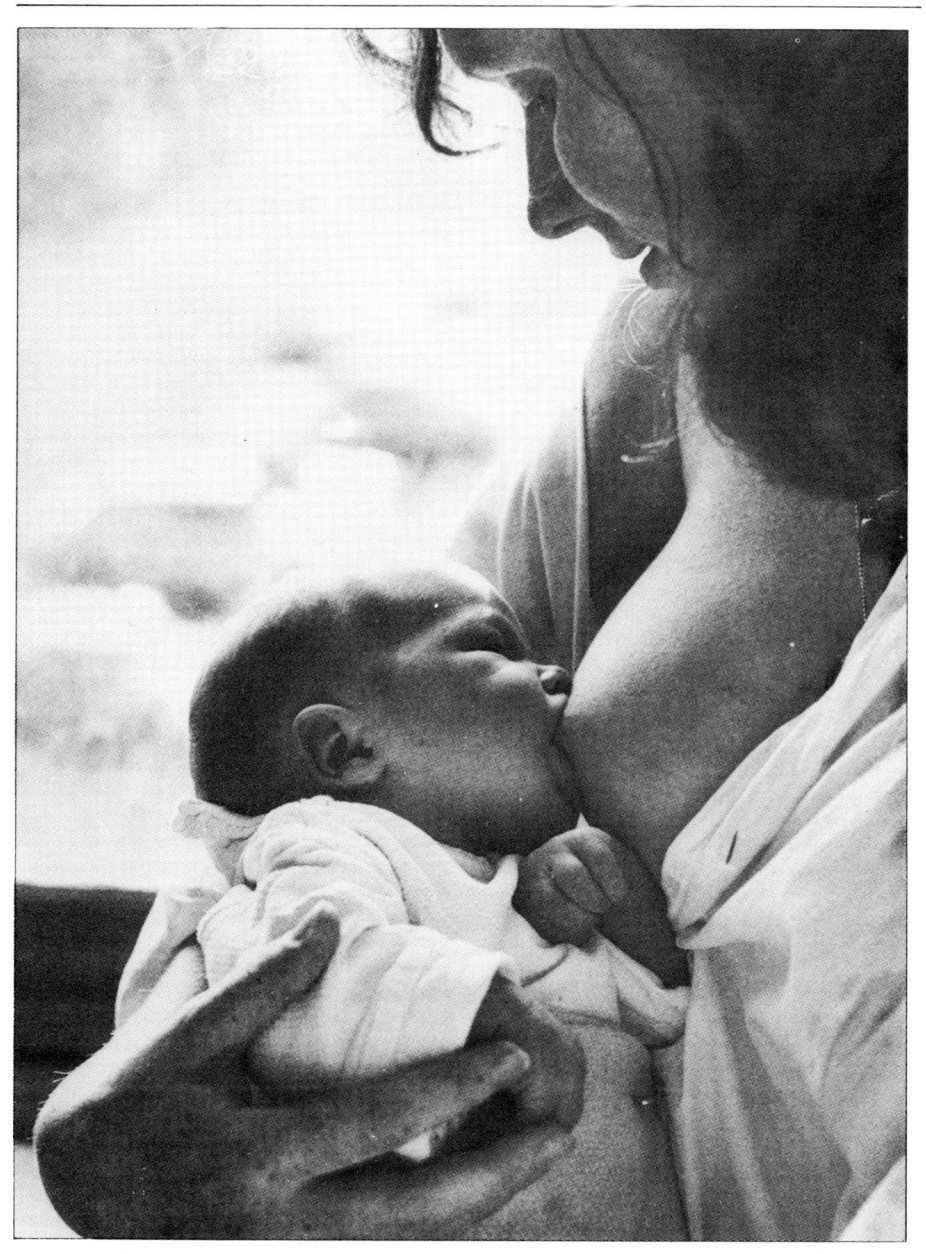

Most women choose to breastfeed their babies, if they can, and more and more continue to feed for longer.

BREAST PUMPS

BREAST PUMPS Usually, there's no need for a breastfeeding mother to use a breast pump, but occasionally there are circumstances where one is required. A breast pump draws off the milk in your breasts in a similar way to a breastfeeding infant. There are different sorts available and they suit different situations. Your hospital will probably have an electric breast pump. Its main use will be to help mothers of pre-term or sick babies to express their milk so that it can be given to their babies by bottle or tube (tiny ill babies sometimes aren't strong enough to suck at the breast). If you are discharged from hospital before your baby for some reason, and you want to continue breastfeeding, you'll perhaps need a breast pump at home. You can hire an electric breast pump from agents who belong to the National Childbirth Trust pump hire scheme. Other pumps are operated by hand, and they can be quite useful for the occasional expressing session. Some women need to express a little milk before a feed because of *engorgement*. You might also like to express milk in advance of a night out to be left for your babysitter to give by bottle. Hand-expressing without a pump can be just as effective – your midwife, health visitor or breastfeeding counsellor will explain how to do it (see *expressing milk*, also Useful Addresses).

BREASTS Your breasts are the human version of mammary glands, designed to secrete milk to feed human babies. During pregnancy, your breasts prepare themselves for this very function, and in a first-time mother the changes to her breasts may be noticed even before she's missed her first period. In the first few weeks of pregnancy, hormones cause much of the fatty tissue on the breasts to be replaced by milk-producing cells and ducts. This, plus an increased blood supply to the breasts often makes the breasts larger and heavier than usual. You may feel tingling sensations at times, and if you haven't had a baby before you'll almost certainly see your nipples are darker in colour and even larger in size (redheads and other fair-skinned types might not notice this). *Montgomery's tubercles* – small spots – also appear on the nipples.

Even if you don't normally wear a bra, you will probably need the comfort and support of one now. Some women find their breasts become very sensitive during pregnancy. If you normally enjoy your breasts being caressed as part of love-making, these sensations may increase – a bonus! Conversely, you might find you need to ask your partner to be extra gentle as the sensation can border on the uncomfortable or even painful. Either way, whatever you feel, it's normal.

There is a school of thought that suggests it's a good idea to prepare your breasts for feeding (by using creams or oils to keep them supple, and expressing *colostrum* which should start being produced in later pregnancy). The newer thinking though, says this isn't necessary, but do it if you feel like it, as it can't do any harm. Washing your breasts every day is important to remove any residues of colostrum, though don't put soap on your nipples, as this can dry them out and leave

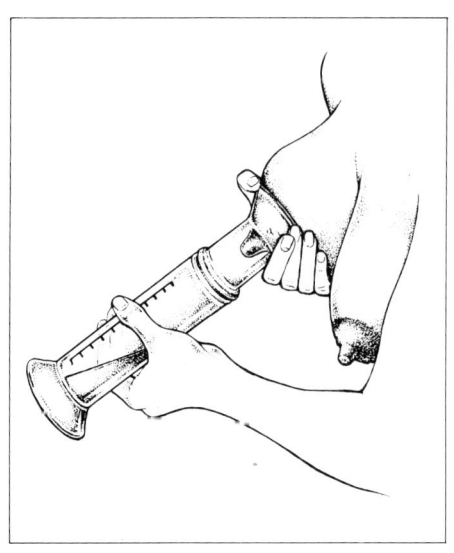

Expressing milk with a hand breast pump.

BREATHING

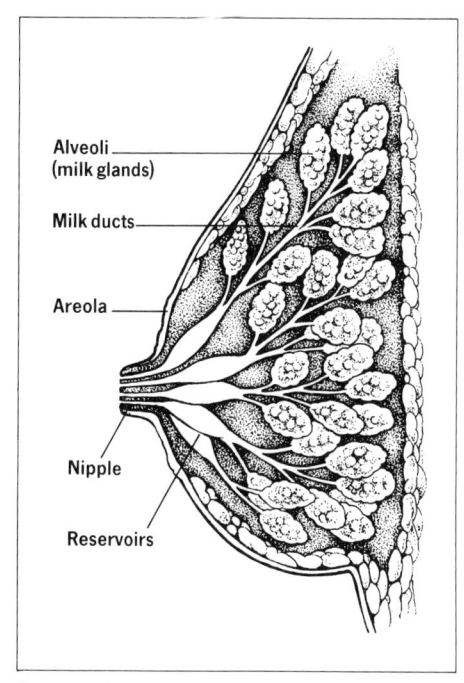

Alveoli (milk glands)
Milk ducts
Areola
Nipple
Reservoirs

Cross-section of the breast.
The milk is produced and stored in the glands (alveoli), and let down through the ducts leading to the nipple. A small amount of milk is stored in the reservoirs behind the nipple.

them sore. The normal nipple secretions of pregnancy should be enough to keep your nipples soft and supple (see *breastfeeding*).

BREAST SHELLS These are sometimes called breast shields. They are small plastic devices with a hole in the centre, where your nipple goes. Their purpose is to draw out flat or inverted nipples to make them a better shape for the baby to *latch on* to for feeding. Worn for short periods during pregnancy they can be effective, though mothers with flat or inverted nipples say the shape of their nipples often improves spontaneously during pregnancy anyway, and during the early days of feeding. Your ante-natal clinic or breastfeeding counsellor will advise you on whether shells would help, and the clinic will usually be able to lend you them when necessary.

BREATHING Many women find that breathing techniques during labour are an excellent way to relieve pain. They particularly enjoy the sense of being in control of their labour, a feeling that drugs can take away completely. Ante-natal classes often deliberately teach different breathing 'levels' to cope with different types of contraction and different levels of pain. This sort of teaching was a great part of *psychoprophylaxis* and in some ways the breathing was seen as a distractor to the pain.

Now, however, the emphasis seems to be changing. Some people feel a rigid breathing formula can be less helpful, and that it can interfere with the woman's ability to listen to her own individual needs in labour. So although breathing can be marvellously helpful, it should be seen as a means of achieving the sort of relaxation labouring women need to have, if they are to concentrate their energies on giving birth, and to be in tune with what their bodies are telling them. If you are as relaxed as you can be, the sort of breathing you need to help you along comes naturally, they say, and you don't need to have learnt all the different patterns. It's true that women who have learnt the 'correct' breathing sometimes find it all flies out the window once things get really going, and women who undergo long and difficult labours may find it ceases to be effective. Yet other women find they manage to hang on to their breathing techniques and by doing so remain in control, because this is something they're really sure of. These women could find an approach based on 'relax, be confident, and make it up as you go along' confusing and untrustworthy. The debate is still at its height, and I imagine the conclusion will be that different approaches suit different women. I suspect, too, that breathing will be seen as a vital part of the relaxation that everyone agrees is helpful to both mother and baby (see *active birth*).

BREATHING DIFFICULTIES Some babies – particularly pre-term ones – have problems with their breathing at birth. Some start breathing by themselves after only a few seconds, and the crisis is over, whereas others need a whiff or two of oxygen. A very few need to be actively resuscitated and in most hospital delivery rooms the right equipment is already present to deal with just such an emergency. Pre-term babies may suffer from *respiratory distress syndrome* which needs special medical and nursing care. A very few babies who have breathing difficulties at birth go on to show evidence of other problems in later infancy or childhood, which is why clinic doctors sometimes ask the routine question 'Did she have any problems breathing at birth?' when carrying out developmental checks.

BREATHLESSNESS If you're breathless, it will probably be towards the end of pregnancy when your expanded uterus is pressing upwards on to your diaphragm and giving your lungs less room to inflate. It's a bit of a nuisance, but if it becomes uncomfortable or even painful, tell your doctor or midwife. Standing or sitting up straight can help sometimes. It may go after *'lightening'* when the baby has dropped down in your pelvis a little. Some women have short attacks of breathlessness in early pregnancy. The cause for this could be hormonal. It's not usually serious, and it goes after the first three months or so, but even so it should be reported to your doctor.

BREECH PRESENTATION Most babies are born in such a way that the head is the presenting part – that is, it's the head that's born first. A baby presenting by the breech is delivered bottom first (or, more rarely, legs first). Until about the 34th or 35th week of pregnancy, the baby may lie in any of several positions – including breech – and he may often change his position. Sometime in those last four to six weeks, however, he 'decides' on a presentation which he sticks to until he is born. In about three cases in every 100, the presentation is breech. It's not ideal; it means the head is born last, which could be dangerous if there's any delay in the second stage, and the other main risk is that the umbilical cord can slip down before the presenting part and become compressed. However, most breech babies are spotted ante-natally and risks known about in advance can usually be averted. Some obstetricians deliver most of 'their' breech babies by caesarean section; others feel quite happy about delivering breech babies vaginally, as long as there don't seem to be any other problems such as prematurity or the baby being small-for-dates. There are arguments for and against both points of view, and if your baby is breech you should have the chance to discuss caesarean and vaginal birth with your consultant. When a breech baby is born vaginally, many consultants use forceps as this can give a controlled, non-delayed second stage. Most specialists prefer the mother of a breech baby to deliver lying down, rather than upright, as they feel the delivery can be controlled more successfully in this position. However, there is a view that a breech baby benefits from the mother being in an upright position, and this again is something you need to discuss before the birth.

During your pregnancy, once it's clear your baby's breech, your doctor may decide to try external cephalic version. This is a manoeuvre that has to be done carefully, by someone skilled in it (mainly to avoid the risk of the placenta separating from the uterine wall). It's an attempt (quite painless, by the way) to change the position of the baby manually to a head first one. It sometimes works, though often the baby won't turn, or else turns right back again later.

For delivery, it might be suggested you have an *epidural*. It takes away the urge to push, so you don't feel the need to bear down too soon in second stage (see *birth position; prolapse of the cord*).

CAESAREAN SECTION

BROW PRESENTATION This is a position of the baby in the uterus. The head is down, but the chin isn't well-flexed (tucked in) and the presenting part of the baby (that is the part that will be born first) is the brow. This is the widest part of the baby's head, and it may be too wide to descend through the pelvis. Unless the fetus is small, and the pelvis is large, the baby is likely to have to be delivered by *caesarean section*.

BUTTERFLY MASK The popular name for chloasma. It's a mild pigmentation of the face – forehead, nose and cheeks, usually – that sometimes affects a women during pregnancy. It fades soon after delivery.

C

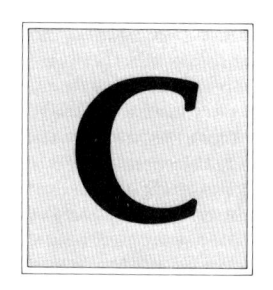

CAESAREAN SECTION The word comes from the Latin word meaning 'to cut' – not because Julius Caesar was a caesarean baby as everyone thinks. It involves the delivery of the baby by cutting through your abdomen into the womb. The baby, membranes and placenta are lifted out, and then you're sewn back up again. The whole thing only takes 40 minutes or so. The cut is usually a 'bikini' cut – low down so that it is covered when the pubic hair regrows.

Some babies are born by elective section, that is, both doctor and mother know in advance that a section is planned. Others are born by *emergency caesarean section*, when the mother has already gone into labour, perhaps because the baby is distressed and needs to be delivered quickly.

You may be advised that you'll need a caesarean section because of *disproportion* – when the size of your baby isn't ideally matched to the size and shape of your pelvis; your baby may be in a less-than-straightforward position for delivery (*breech*, for instance); he may not be growing well and the strain of a vaginal delivery may be thought too much for him, or it may be necessary for him to be born before term in order to give him a chance of surviving, and *induction* is not usually used for mothers expecting babies who may be very tiny and weak. If the subject of a caesarean section comes up, make sure you have the chance to discuss it fully with your consultant and also, if you can, the sister on the post-natal ward who'll be looking after you. If you'd like to see your baby just as soon

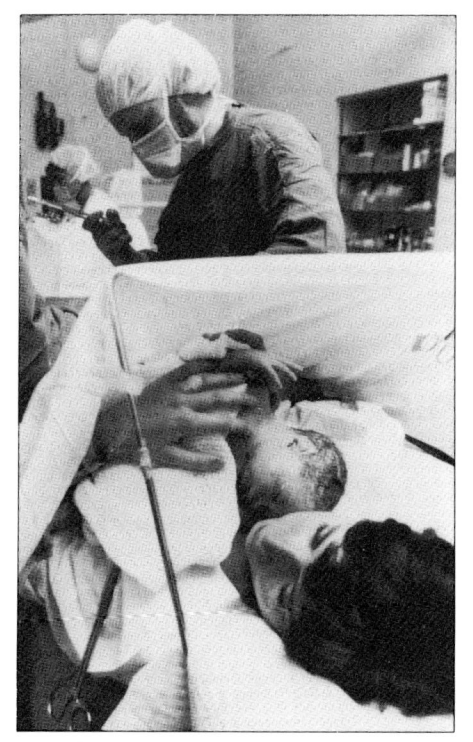

You can hold your baby immediately after a Caesarean birth if all is well.

29

as you regain consciousness, and to start breastfeeding as soon as is practicable, then do say so. These days, keeping mother and baby apart after a section for 24 or even 48 hours is rarely done (unless there are exceptional circumstances), but it's worth having your mind put at rest on these points.

If you'd like to be conscious during the birth, many hospitals will perform a caesarean section under an *epidural* anaesthetic. This takes away the sensation of pain while you are being cut and stitched, but leaves you and your baby in a good condition afterwards (a general anaesthetic can make you woozy and nauseous, and has certain risks of its own). This means that you will be able to see and touch your baby straightaway, as after a normal delivery. Also, some hospitals allow the father to be present during a caesarean done under epidural anaesthetic.

Any surgery with anaesthesia is potentially dangerous, but caesarean sections are among the most safe and routine of operations. However, from your point of view a section is a surgical operation, albeit one with very positive results, on the whole, and you'll need help, support and rest afterwards. Take everything gently at first: you'll need help positioning the baby whether you are breast or bottle feeding, for instance (for sympathetic support after a caesarean section, see Useful Addresses).

Between 10 and 12 per cent of babies in this country are born by caesarean section, and the rate has risen over the past few years, something which has been the subject of much discussion recently. It has been suggested that obstetricians are too 'knife-happy', for a variety of reasons. Some say that doctors nowadays prefer to do a section rather than a potentially tricky forceps delivery. Others point to the fact that a large proportion of breech babies are born by section these days. The debate continues, though we should all be concerned in case the UK section rate creeps up to join the United States' one (in some centres 40 per cent), where it seems to be a result of 'defensive obstetrics' – the doctor feeling he ought to take every possible precaution against parents suing him for

negligence. If you have one section, it doesn't have to mean that subsequent babies can't be born vaginally. This depends on the reason for the section (see *trial of labour*).

CALCIUM An essential constituent of anyone's *diet*, calcium is particularly important during pregnancy, as it helps form healthy teeth and bones. You need more calcium in pregnancy. Now research suggests it can help prevent *pre-eclampsia*, especially if you drink whole milk (which contains Vitamin D, needed for the absorption of calcium). Other sources: cheese, nuts and green vegetables.

CAPUT *(ká-putt)* A very temporary swelling on the head of a newborn baby. It's merely a result of pressure from the cervix during labour. It can appear on the face or on the back instead, whichever part has been born first.

CARPAL TUNNEL SYNDROME This is a side-effect of pregnancy experienced by women. It tends to occur in the last few months, and it's a result of fluid retention. The fluid builds up in your wrists and presses down on the nerves there, causing tingling, even numb sensations. It can happen at any time, but a lot of women notice it after a night's sleep. You can help to ease it by raising your arm above your head for a few minutes, which allows the fluid to drain away.

CARTIOCOGRAPHY This is sometimes known as CTG. It's a method – carried out by machine – that measures the heart rate of a baby, either during pregnancy or during labour (see *fetal monitor*).

CASTOR OIL Castor oil is a laxative. Traditionally it's used as a way of getting an already overdue labour to start. The idea is that the resultant bowel action triggers off a sympathetic muscular response in the uterus.

Castor oil is revolting to take (though you could mix it with orange juice to make it more palatable) and you might find the laxative effect a bit strong, but it hasn't been shown to be harmful. It won't work if labour wasn't about to start anyway, but you could just hasten things along by a few hours by taking it.

CATHETER *(ká-thuta)* A long fine tube used in medical treatment for various reasons. During labour it might be used to relieve your bladder (the midwife inserts it – quite painlessly – into your urethra, which is the exit point for your urine). Usually, however, you won't need this done as you will be able to pass urine quite easily.

CAUL If the waters round the baby in the womb have been left intact until the end of labour, or if they haven't broken spontaneously, the new baby may be born with the membranes still over his face. When this happens he's said to be born in a caul. The membranes are always removed immediately so the baby can breathe. It's rare, these days, for a baby to be born in a caul, as the waters are almost always broken artificially if they don't 'go' by themselves. At one time, it was thought to be a sort of lucky omen to be born in a caul: Charles Dickens' David Copperfield was born like this, and his caul was sold to a fisherman as a protection against drowning! (see *artificial rupture of the membranes*).

CEPHALHAEMATOMA *(kefal-heema-toma)* This is a swelling that might develop on a baby's scalp a day or so after birth (sometimes after a difficult delivery). It's actually a sort of bruise: a collection of blood over one of the bones of the skull, and it's caused by friction between the mother's pelvis and the baby's skull. Although it can make the shape of the head look worryingly odd, the blood is absorbed over a few weeks and the swelling subsides, leaving a perfectly normal shaped head. No treatment is necessary.

CHILD BENEFIT

CEPHALIC *(kefálic)* The best way for a baby to be born – a cephalic presentation means 'head first'. The opposite is *breech*.

CERVICAL EROSION This is a relatively common condition. It happens when the normal skin on the outside of the *cervix* is replaced by an overgrowth of skin from the inside of the cervix. It's normally left untreated during pregnancy, as it often cures itself. The main problem associated with it is that it can cause some slight bleeding, particularly after intercourse, and this can be confused with the sort of slight bleeding that can herald the start of a threatened miscarriage.

CERVICAL SMEAR TEST See *smear test*.

CERVIX The neck of the womb or uterus, linking the vagina and the womb. In pregnancy it becomes softer and more swollen than before. Towards the end of pregnancy it becomes even softer, in preparation for the dilatation (opening and stretching) required during birth – this is the so-called 'ripening' of the cervix midwives and doctors talk about. During labour the muscular contractions gradually open up the cervix more and more, so that the baby can pass through the birth canal. Progress in labour is expressed in terms of the number of centimetres dilated – it has to open to about 10 cms or five fingers to let the baby through. Dilatation of the cervix tends to take less time for a second or subsequent baby.

CHILD BENEFIT Parents of all children under the age of 16 are entitled to a cash benefit, the same amount for each child, normally paid every four weeks. You make your initial claim at any social security office and cash the slips from the benefit book at a post office. You will need to send your child's birth certificate with your completed claim form (this is of course returned to you). If you are a single parent, you can claim a separate rate on a different form.

CHLOASMA

CHLOASMA *(kl-o-áz-ma)* See *butterfly mask*.

CHOOSING A HOSPITAL Most women these days have their babies in hospital, and if this is what you are planning, you may have a choice, especially if you live in an urban area. Theoretically, you can have your baby in any hospital with a maternity unit, but some hospitals have a 'catchment area' policy which excludes women living outside the local area. If you have a real choice, then think about where you would like to have your baby before you see your GP to have your pregnancy confirmed. Ask women who have recently had babies what their experience has been; local organisations (such as the National Childbirth Trust) may be able to help with recent information on hospital practices and routines. Your GP himself may have knowledge, too, and he may be able to help you decide which consultant you would like to be 'under', as this too can make some difference. You can always change your mind about where you want to have your baby during pregnancy, though it's not always very easy to arrange, and the bureaucracy doesn't always co-operate efficiently. If you move house any distance, though, obviously you have to change hospitals. Basically, what you are looking for when you choose a hospital is flexibility on the part of staff – and that goes whether you want a high-tech birth or active birth or whatever – and a hospital policy that takes into account individual needs and wishes, ante-natally, during the birth, and post-natally on the wards. A reputation for long waits at the ante-natal clinic means a minus point, too (see *hospital birth*).

CHORION VILLUS SAMPLING. A new technique – also known as chorion biopsy – whose pioneers hope will eventually lead to the end of *amniocentesis* in many cases, with its consequent risks and disadvantages. In early pregnancy, tiny fibres called chorionic villii attach the fetus to the uterus wall. At about eight weeks of pregnancy, one of these fibres can be taken out via the cervix and analysed. The information given on analysis includes what sex the fetus is, plus important genetic data leading to a diagnosis of certain hereditary and chromosomal disorders. At present, chorion biopsy is available in a very few centres in this country, and the applications of the technique are still being carefully studied. Results so far are hopeful, but it's not yet known for certain just how safe, or otherwise, it is for a normal fetus. Routine testing – if it ever arrives – must be several years away.

CHORIONIC GONADOTROPHIN *(koreeónic gonad-o-trófin)* See *HCG*.

CHROMOSOME *(kró-mo-some)* Every normal human cell contains 46 chromosomes arranged as pairs. These are the containers of genetic information that govern our inherited characteristics. At conception, the only two human cells which have 23 chromosomes – the egg from the female and the spermatozoon from the male – unite to form one 46-chromosome cell, and set the blueprint for a new life.

CIRCUMCISION This is an operation involving the removal of the loose skin (or foreskin) at the end of a boy's penis. It's done for religious reasons in this country when the parents wish it, and occasionally for medical reasons. There's no real reason to believe circumcision has any general health benefit.

CLEFT LIP/PALATE This is a defect that happens while the baby is still in the womb. The two halves of the palate (roof of the mouth) and/or the upper lip fail to fuse, and the baby is born with an opening in his palate, and if he has a cleft lip as well, the upper lip has a large opening in it, too. The main problem at first is feeding, but with support and the right sort of advice, this can be managed. Depending on the degree of the cleft, some mothers manage to breastfeed though in many cases, bottle feeding, perhaps with expressed breast milk, is the only solution (probably with a specially-shaped teat). Surgery to repair the cleft is almost always extremely successful, and the majority of children go on to have no further problems at all, once corrective surgery is over.

CLOTHES FOR BABY Many parents get presents of clothing for a newborn baby but not all of it is very practical. For the first few months all a baby needs is a few stretchsuits (at least six) which he can wear day and night; two or three cardigans or matinee jackets; a couple of shawls; one or two hats; one or two pairs of mittens; nappies, plastic pants; about six vests. Winter babies may need some outer garments for wearing in the pram, but being wrapped up in a shawl, and being under blankets, perhaps with a hat on too, should be enough on top of his ordinary clothes. Make sure everything you buy is machine-washable and easy to put on and off – this is of course one of the beauties of stretchsuits, as they open down the front and down each leg, making nappy changing and dressing and undressing so much easier. I've heard mothers say they make babies look like overstuffed sausages – true, but the traditional alternative, long white nightgowns, need ironing (horrors), they ride up over the baby's tummy, and they need to be pulled off over the head (see *equipment for baby*).

CLOTHES FOR MOTHER See *maternity wear*.

COLOSTRUM The fluid produced in the breasts during the second half of pregnancy and in the first few days after the birth of the baby before the milk comes in. It's highly valuable for the new baby as it contains *antibodies* as well as a very concentrated amount of nutrients. If you aren't sure whether you want to breastfeed, it would be worth giving your baby colostrum, and then switching to the bottle if this is what you would prefer.

It's sometimes suggested that pregnant mothers express colostrum during pregnancy, but it hasn't been shown that this has any bearing on successful breastfeeding, and we really don't know if doing this means the baby will get less colostrum as a result. My own feeling is that it's probably not worth doing unless seeing the colostrum 'proves' to you that you will be able to breastfeed. Even so, many women find they can't express colostrum because they don't have the knack of expressing, not because there's nothing there.

If you find you leak colostrum during pregnancy, possibly from around the sixth month, wash off the dried crusts that result with warm water – not soap, as it's too drying.

COMMUNITY HEALTH COUNCIL (in Scotland, Local Health Council). This is the consumer's voice in the National Health Service. Apart from a paid secretary, CHCs are comprised of volunteer representatives from local organisations and they report to the District Health Authority. If you need information about health services in your area, a good place to start looking is the CHC. Contact the secretary (the number for your CHC will be in the telephone book).

COMMUNITY MIDWIFE The community midwife's main work is outside hospital, though of course she will almost certainly have worked in a hospital in the past. Part of her role is to look after the ante-natal care of women intending to have their babies at home, or women choosing shared care at their GP's surgery or at the health centre. She may well take preparation classes for labour and birth at the same place. She will also deliver you if you have your baby at home. Many community midwifes may also deliver babies in hospital, for women who have arranged '*domino*' deliveries, or other short stay options.

COMPLICATIONS OF PREGNANCY

The community midwife visits mothers at home for at least 10 days, and up to 28 days, after the birth (see *midwife*).

COMPLICATIONS OF PREGNANCY
Most pregnancies progress perfectly straightforwardly, and the major purpose of *ante-natal care* is to spot those few pregnancies that develop problems – complications – of one sort or another, which may have an effect on the unborn baby's health or on the delivery. Among the less uncommon complications are a rise in *blood pressure; pre-eclampsia; bleeding.*

CONCEPTION
Conception happens when a sperm from a man fertilises an egg (ovum) from a woman. It's actually a complex biochemical process and a truly miraculous one. Only one egg per month (usually that is) is ripened and released by the ovaries (this is called *ovulation*), but several hundred million sperm are produced by the testes and released at every ejaculation. Even so, only one sperm fuses with the egg (except in cases of non-identical twins and triplets and so on, when more than one egg is fertilised by the same number of sperm) and this happens when the egg is in the *fallopian tube* during its journey to the womb or uterus. In the vast

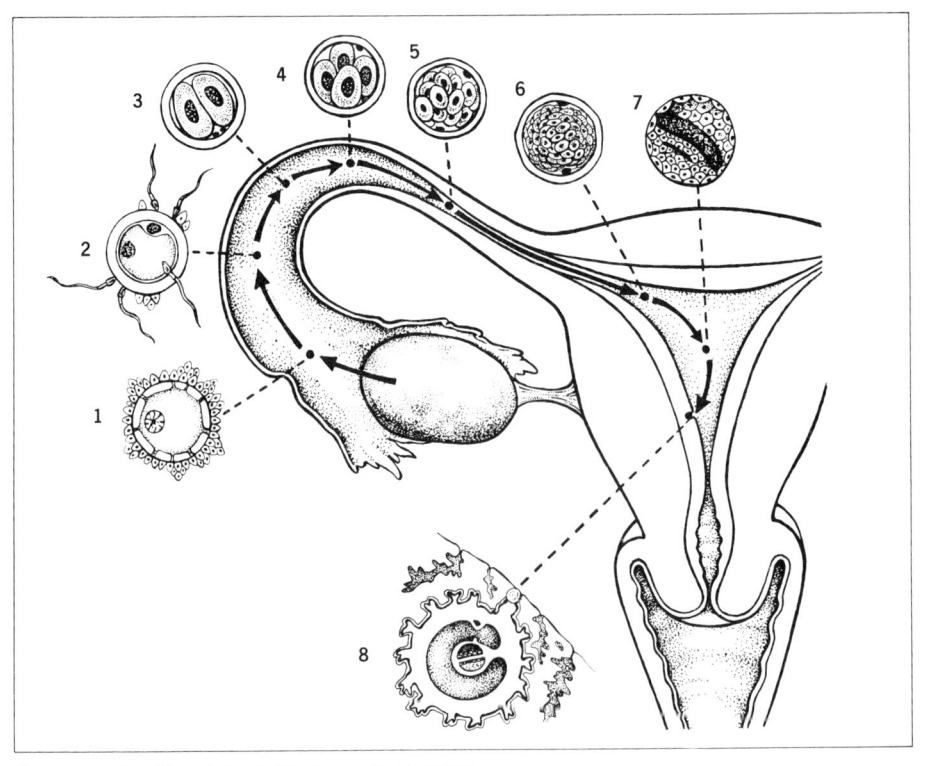

Pregnancy begins with ovulation, fertilisation, and implantation.
1 The egg is released from the ovary at ovulation. 2 The egg is fertilised by a sperm. 3 The sperm and egg fuse.
4 Cell division begins and continues 5 and 6 as the fertilised egg is wafted along the fallopian tube.
7 The fertilised egg finally reaches the uterus and embeds in the lining 8.

majority of cases conception takes place as a result of sexual intercourse at or around the time of ovulation.

Conception can, and does, take place outside the body, as with so-called test-tube babies, which doctors more correctly term 'in vitro fertilisation' (IVF) meaning 'fertilisation within glass', where sperm and ovum are fused in the laboratory. With *AID* and *AIH*, fertilisation results after the sperm are produced separately to intercourse, and then placed within the woman's cervical canal.

CONFINEMENT A word which refers to the period of labour and delivery and the *puerperium*.

CONGENITAL A congenital abnormality or handicap is one that is present when the baby is born – it doesn't develop as a result of birth injury, or later as a result of illness or disease. It need not necessarily be a hereditary problem.

CONGENITAL DISLOCATION OF THE HIP (CDH) A not very uncommon condition present at birth, when the head of the baby's thigh bone doesn't sit neatly in the hip socket. Routine examination for CDH takes place shortly after a baby is born, when the doctor gently manipulates the baby's legs and checks for normal movement. In this way, many babies with CDH are detected soon enough for the defect to be treated by a splint or a special plaster. Some babies with a mild degree of dislocation can be put into double nappies for a few weeks, and the condition cures itself. If left untreated, CDH can lead to a limp.

CONSTIPATION This is often a side-effect of pregnancy. The higher levels of hormone in your body cause everything to slow down and slacken, and that can mean your digestive system works more slowly than before. The result can be an increased tendency to

CONTRACTIONS

constipation, which in turn can lead to *piles*. But if your diet is high in *fibre* you should be far less likely to suffer from this complaint. As at other times, laxatives should only be used after you have tried drinking lots of extra fluid and upped your fibre intake (and do see your doctor before you dose yourself with laxatives). If you find your iron tablets make you constipated, tell your clinic and they can give you another brand to try.

It's normal not to want to open your bowels for a few days after your baby's born, but if you're staying in hospital longer than this you may find that standard hospital food doesn't give you the high fibre levels you may have got used to, and you may end up constipated. The solution is to ask friends and relatives to bring in fruit and, if you can stand the taste, bran.

CONSULTANT The consultant is a doctor, who heads a medical team, in a hospital. In a large maternity unit, you could easily have three, four, five or even more consultant obstetricians; in a small unit there may be only one. When you book in to your chosen hospital at the start of pregnancy, you'll be assigned to a consultant and he will be nominally in charge of your ante-natal care, delivery and post-natal care. If everything goes normally, you might not even see him, as consultants tend to concentrate their time and skills on the more problematic cases. However, if you have a query about hospital policy, or if you want something a bit 'different', the consultant is the person to discuss it with.

CONTRACEPTION See *family planning*.

CONTRACTIONS Regular contractions are one of the symptoms of labour, and they are needed to push the baby out of the uterus, through the birth canal and into the world. The uterus itself is made up of muscle, and during labour contractions, the muscle fibres contract – they become shorter and thicker. At

35

CONVULSIONS

the end of a contraction they relax, but they don't go right back to the size they were. The result is that as labour progresses, the contractions cause the uterus to become smaller, so there's less room for the baby and she is literally 'squeezed out'. The contractions also pull up and dilate the cervix, thinning out the tissue, so the opening gradually enlarges until it's wide enough for the baby to descend down the birth canal.

In many women, contractions start off as a sort of tightening, something like a dull sort of period pain, becoming stronger and more frequent as labour progresses. They start very gently, then gradually build up to a peak before dying away again. At the end of the first stage they may last well over a minute, and be happening every two or three minutes. During the second stage, each contraction may follow on closely from the previous one, though you always get some sort of a pause between them. Every labour is different, however, and you may experience quite different lengths and frequency and still be perfectly normal. Almost everyone experiences a gradual build-up of contractions, though, and when they become more frequent and longer over a period it's a sign that everything's progressing as it should.

Contractions have been likened to waves in their shape, and many women find that quite an accurate image. Most women find contractions are painful some of the time, but this sensation of *pain* is experienced very differently. Sometimes it may be no more than a twinge or an ache; at the other end of the spectrum some women find the pain to be quite unbearable.

During pregnancy, you may feel *Braxton-Hicks contractions*, which are usually painless, and are part of the uterus' preparation for labour.

CONVULSIONS ('FITS') Any convulsions during pregnancy should be taken very seriously indeed. In later pregnancy they can be a symptom of *eclampsia*, now fortunately a rare condition as the signs of *pre-eclampsia* are almost always spotted and acted upon ante-natally. Convulsions in a newborn baby are cause for concern as well, though very often the cause can be identified and dealt with without any long-term ill-effects noted. One cause of a baby's convulsions, for example, is low blood-sugar level (*hypoglycaemia*). Once diagnosed (by a blood test) the treatment is quick and effective: sugar given orally or by drip, and normal breast or bottle feeding.

CO-OPERATION CARD This is a card on which is recorded all the important information about you and your pregnancy that you keep yourself. It's actually meant to be a sort of handy information package between the hospital ante-natal clinic and the family doctor who is sharing your care, if that's the sort of ante-natal care you have opted for. When you have a hospital ante-natal appointment, the staff note down on your co-op card things like your blood pressure, the result of your urine test, your weight and anything else that's been checked, together with any comments. Your GP or midwife do the same when you see them. Ask about anything you don't understand on your card: it's pointless getting anxious because you can't decipher a doctor's squiggle, or because some of the terminology is unknown to you.

CORPUS LUTEUM Literally, this translates as 'yellow body'. Within the ovary the immature eggs are contained in protective cavities called follicles. Each month, one of the follicles ruptures and an egg is released. After the egg has been released (that is, after *ovulation*), the follicle develops into the corpus luteum (which is, in fact, yellowish in colour, hence the name). If conception doesn't happen, the corpus luteum simply dies away. If on the other hand conception takes place, the corpus luteum secretes a hormone (progesterone) that sustains the pregnancy until the placenta takes over hormone production at around the 14th week.

CRAMP Cramp, particularly in your legs and feet, is quite common in pregnancy, usually occurring at night. It's been postulated that it is caused by a salt or calcium deficiency so you could check your diet if you're troubled by it. Modern diets aren't likely to go short of salt, however, and calcium intake can be increased by drinking more milk, though calcium supplements can be prescribed.

If you get cramp, try pulling your toes up towards you while pushing your heel forwards. Rubbing your leg vigorously can also help.

CROWNING The moment during delivery when the baby's head appears out of the birth canal.

CRYING BABY All new babies cry. Some cry more than others. Some even seem to spend most of the day and night crying. The problem is that as parents you can feel so helpless when faced with a baby who won't stop crying. Is she genuinely ill? In pain? Hungry? Tired? Not tired enough? Bored? Cold? Hot? Wet? Dirty? Overstimulated? A baby who cries incessantly without you being able to comfort her certainly needs to be checked over medically to rule out any organic cause for the distress. (And distress it is. Babies don't cry for the hell of it, or because they're spoilt, or because they like to see you running round in circles.) In the vast majority of cases the baby is pronounced fit and well, and you're back to square one. Always treat a very new baby's crying as caused by hunger in the first instance, even if you've just fed her. If she's hungry, a healthy baby will suck (though she may need to be calmed down by rocking, singing or whatever before she can be in a state to feed). Bottle fed babies are sometimes thirsty rather than hungry, particularly in summer or in a hot hospital ward. Lots of babies cry because they need the reassurance and security of a cuddle. Some babies seem to need this all the time, and their parents have found the solution to the constant crying by simply carrying the baby close to them at all times, and even sleeping with them at night. It's as if babies like these hate the thought that as soon as they are quiet, they'll be put down in a cot, away from the human contact and warmth they thrive on. The trouble is that our modern lifestyle doesn't find it easy to accommodate a baby in constant close contact; you do need a baby sling, a relaxed attitude to housework, supportive friends and family – and perhaps a much more baby-centred outlook than most of us want to aspire to.

Remember that as time goes on, whatever you do, you and your baby will develop a more understanding relationship, and the crying almost always gets better, mainly because you learn to assess more accurately what's causing it. If the crying gets you down, don't hesitate to look for help and support from within or outside your family. Health visitors, breastfeeding counsellors, midwives, post-natal supporters, kind neighbours – almost anyone with experience of young babies knows the strain that even one evening's crying can bring, and they will be sympathetic. One final point: breastfed babies sometimes react by crying to something that doesn't agree with them in their mother's diet. Experiment, if you like, particularly by cutting out cows' milk and cows' milk products from your diet. If you make long-term changes to your eating, though, you may need vitamin and mineral supplements, and/or advice on the rest of your diet. Again, see your health visitor, doctor or dietician.

CYST A structure filled with fluid and covered with membrane. It can appear almost anywhere in the body. Women can develop ovarian cysts on the ovary. They can go undiagnosed for some time and may not cause any obvious problems. However, if an ovarian cyst is discovered during pregnancy it's often removed surgically. This is to rule out completely the chance that the cyst may obstruct the growing pregnancy or the progress of labour, and to avoid the possibility of torsion, when the cyst starts to twist, which would be extremely painful.

CYSTITIS

CYSTITIS An inflammation of the bladder, which can make passing urine quite painful. It can sometimes be cleared up quite quickly by drinking lots of water or an alkaline drink such as lemon barley to flush the infection out, and if this isn't effective your doctor may prescribe antibiotics (remind him you're pregnant). Once you've had cystitis you'll know the warning signs: slight stinging when you pass urine, a need to pass urine frequently, perhaps a dull pain. Stop it getting worse by drinking as much water as you can, and help prevent further attacks by wearing cotton underwear, stockings rather than tights (or crotchless tights).

D

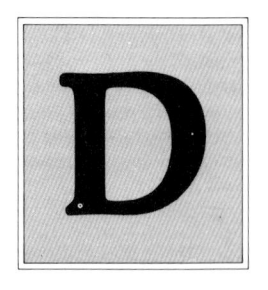

CUTTING THE CORD While in the womb the *umbilical cord* is what links the baby with the placenta. After birth, it needs to be severed at some point (there are no nerves in the cord so this is not painful for mother and baby). Standard practice is to clamp and cut the cord almost immediately after the baby is born, usually within the first two minutes or so. The justification for this when the baby appears healthy and not in need of any immediate attention is not very great. It does allow the midwife to wrap the baby up to keep her warm, and to wipe her down a bit, but wiping can be done with or without the cord attached, and a healthy baby only needs the warmth of her mother's arms and body in the first minutes after birth, to stop her from getting chilled. There are advantages in leaving the cord unclamped: as long as the baby is attached to the placenta she is able to get oxygen even if she isn't yet breathing with her lungs. The placenta and cord continue to function until the cord stops pulsating, and until this point the baby is receiving valuable oxygenated blood even if she isn't breathing normally. Many midwives are starting to feel happier about leaving the moment of clamping the cord until the cord stops pulsating (usually a matter of minutes), and there is a school of thought that feels it's gentler to allow nature to take its course in this way, to give a more gradual changeover from being linked to the mother to being a separate individual. If you'd like to be given your baby to hold immediately, before the cord is cut, ask in advance.

D & C Dilatation and curettage, or, as it is commonly known a 'scrape'. This is a fairly routine operation, done under general anaesthetic in hospital. The dilatation is the opening of the cervix in order to reach the inside of the uterus, which is then scraped with a curette, a sort of long surgical spoon, to remove the lining of the uterus. D & C is sometimes done after miscarriage, to make sure there are no products of conception remaining, and it's sometimes done to help a diagnosis of infertility. After childbirth, it can be done in the case of *retained placenta*.

DANGERS TO AVOID One of the most recently publicised dangers to avoid when you're pregnant is contracting *rubella*. Other dangers include contact with toxic chemicals – possible in certain occupations. You should also avoid X-rays and taking *drugs* that aren't prescribed by your doctor. Nicotine and *alcohol* are potentially very harmful to your unborn baby, too (see *smoking*).

DATING THE PREGNANCY The most usual way of dating a pregnancy, at least in the first instance, is to work out 40 weeks from the first day of the last menstrual period. Another common way is to add 7 days and 9 calendar months to that date which gives more or less

DEEP TRANSVERSE ARREST

January OCTOBER	1 2 3 4 5 6 7 8 9 10 11 12 13 14 15 16 17 18 19 20 21 22 23 24 25 26 27 28 29 30 31	January
	8 9 10 11 12 13 14 15 16 17 18 19 20 21 22 23 24 25 26 27 28 29 30 31 1 2 3 4 5 6 7	NOVEMBER
February NOVEMBER	1 2 3 4 5 6 7 8 9 10 11 12 13 14 15 16 17 18 19 20 21 22 23 24 25 26 27 28	February
	8 9 10 11 12 13 14 15 16 17 18 19 20 21 22 23 24 25 26 27 28 29 30 1 2 3 4 5	DECEMBER
March DECEMBER	1 2 3 4 5 6 7 8 9 10 11 12 13 14 15 16 17 18 19 20 21 22 23 24 25 26 27 28 29 30 31	March
	6 7 8 9 10 11 12 13 14 15 16 17 18 19 20 21 22 23 24 25 26 27 28 29 30 31 1 2 3 4 5	JANUARY
April JANUARY	1 2 3 4 5 6 7 8 9 10 11 12 13 14 15 16 17 18 19 20 21 22 23 24 25 26 27 28 29 30	April
	6 7 8 9 10 11 12 13 14 15 16 17 18 19 20 21 22 23 24 25 26 27 28 29 30 31 1 2 3 4	FEBRUARY
May FEBRUARY	1 2 3 4 5 6 7 8 9 10 11 12 13 14 15 16 17 18 19 20 21 22 23 24 25 26 27 28 29 30 31	May
	5 6 7 8 9 10 11 12 13 14 15 16 17 18 19 20 21 22 23 24 25 26 27 28 1 2 3 4 5 6 7	MARCH
June MARCH	1 2 3 4 5 6 7 8 9 10 11 12 13 14 15 16 17 18 19 20 21 22 23 24 25 26 27 28 29 30	June
	8 9 10 11 12 13 14 15 16 17 18 19 20 21 22 23 24 25 26 27 28 29 30 31 1 2 3 4 5 6	APRIL
July APRIL	1 2 3 4 5 6 7 8 9 10 11 12 13 14 15 16 17 18 19 20 21 22 23 24 25 26 27 28 29 30 31	July
	7 8 9 10 11 12 13 14 15 16 17 18 19 20 21 22 23 24 25 26 27 28 29 30 1 2 3 4 5 6 7	MAY
August MAY	1 2 3 4 5 6 7 8 9 10 11 12 13 14 15 16 17 18 19 20 21 22 23 24 25 26 27 28 29 30 31	August
	8 9 10 11 12 13 14 15 16 17 18 19 20 21 22 23 24 25 26 27 28 29 30 31 1 2 3 4 5 6 7	JUNE
September JUNE	1 2 3 4 5 6 7 8 9 10 11 12 13 14 15 16 17 18 19 20 21 22 23 24 25 26 27 28 29 30	September
	8 9 10 11 12 13 14 15 16 17 18 19 20 21 22 23 24 25 26 27 28 29 30 1 2 3 4 5 6 7	JULY
October JULY	1 2 3 4 5 6 7 8 9 10 11 12 13 14 15 16 17 18 19 20 21 22 23 24 25 26 27 28 29 30 31	October
	8 9 10 11 12 13 14 15 16 17 18 19 20 21 22 23 24 25 26 27 28 29 30 31 1 2 3 4 5 6 7	AUGUST
November AUGUST	1 2 3 4 5 6 7 8 9 10 11 12 13 14 15 16 17 18 19 20 21 22 23 24 25 26 27 28 29 30	November
	8 9 10 11 12 13 14 15 16 17 18 19 20 21 22 23 24 25 26 27 28 29 30 31 1 2 3 4 5 6	SEPTEMBER
December SEPTEMBER	1 2 3 4 5 6 7 8 9 10 11 12 13 14 15 16 17 18 19 20 21 22 23 24 25 26 27 28 29 30 31	December
	7 8 9 10 11 12 13 14 15 16 17 18 19 20 21 22 23 24 25 26 27 28 29 30 1 2 3 4 5 6 7	OCTOBER

Your expected date of delivery can be found by looking on the upper lines of the chart for the first day of your last menstrual period. Your estimated date of delivery, EDD, is below it.

the same result. When there's some confusion about this, or when it isn't known (for instance, if a mother has become pregnant while breastfeeding and hasn't actually started regular periods again, or if she's conceived while on the Pill), experienced midwives and doctors can make accurate guesses from other signs, such as the size of the uterus, when the mother first felt fetal movements, when the fetal heart can be heard. For confirmation of dates, *ultrasound* scans are now widely used. This gives the size of the fetus, and if two scans are taken, the rate of growth can be assessed, and this again can pinpoint dates. Even so, scans can be one or two weeks out (either way), and if you have an irregular menstrual cycle, using your last period as a guide can be unreliable. It's important to have as accurate an idea as possible of when the baby is due, however, not just because it's good to be prepared, but because it's helpful to know your baby is developing at the right rate for the age of gestation.

DEATH IN CHILDBIRTH Very, very rare these days. We have come such a long way in the last two or three generations; before that the statistics were very grim indeed. Doctors did not accept the evidence for the way infections can be transmitted from one person to another, and women died in their thousands from post-childbirth fever, the scourge of the 'lying-in' hospitals of the last century. Nowadays, better general health, ante-natal care, blood transfusions, the prompt dealing with infection, have been among the main reasons for the almost total safety of childbirth today. The risk these days is tiny.

DECIDUA The special lining of the womb during early pregnancy (see *endometrium*).

DEEP TRANSVERSE ARREST This is a complication of labour, and it happens when a baby who has been in an *occipito-posterior*

DELIVERY ROOM

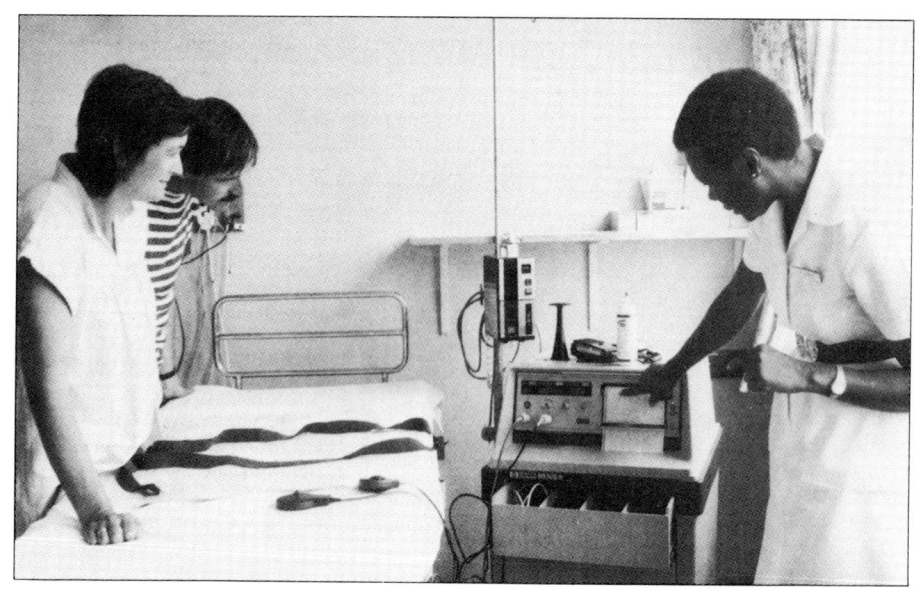

Ask to visit the delivery room during your pregnancy, so you know what to expect when you go in to have your baby.

position – that is with the back of his head towards your spine – rotates and gets stuck halfway round. The head becomes arrested in the pelvis, facing sideways. This almost invariably means you need help in getting your baby born, and a doctor may decide to try turning the head manually, or to use *forceps* or a *ventouse*, to put the baby's head in a better position. Deep transverse arrest is also termed mid-cavity arrest.

DELIVERY ROOM This is the room in hospital where you'll have your baby. It's sometimes called the *birthing room*. In some units, you are transferred to the delivery room from the labour ward; in others you stay in the same place from the time you are admitted. It's a good idea to see the delivery room before you go into labour; if you aren't attending hospital ante-natal classes where a visit is already scheduled, ask during an ante-natal appointment if someone can show you it. It has to be said that some – most – delivery rooms aren't welcoming in appearance. There may be white-tiled walls, harsh lighting; obstetric aids such as the instrument trolley, the fetal monitor and lithotomy stirrups may be well in evidence. The delivery couch may be narrow and high and totally unlike a normal bed. There may not even be a window to let in the outside world. I think those units which are trying to re-think their delivery rooms with rocking chairs, floor cushions, wallpaper and curtains and so on, while trying to keep medical equipment as unobtrusive as possible, need to be encouraged. The place of birth is important: warm colours, homely touches and an unclinical atmosphere can help a woman feel relaxed and welcomed. However, it's the people who really matter, and it's been said by many that no amount of flowery wallpaper will make up for staff who ignore a woman's wishes in labour. And having said that, the standard delivery room, white tiles and all, can be the setting for loving, happy births attended by caring involved staff.

40

DEVELOPMENT OF FETUS

DEMAND FEEDING If you want to breastfeed, then the only sure way to success is to demand feed. It's an unfortunate phrase, really, as it reinforces the outdated notion of crosspatch newborns driving their poor demented mothers to distraction by these (unreasonable) demands for food! But a tiny baby's demands are the same as his needs, and his needs in the early days include having breast milk irregularly, frequently and at any time of the day or night. If you don't feed a newborn baby on demand, and instead try to keep him to a three- or four-hourly schedule, you may find your breast milk supply doesn't get well-established. This is because breast milk is produced as a direct response to your baby's sucking and feeding. Once you and your baby are well-established as a nursing couple, and this can take some weeks, you can nudge your baby into some sort of predictability if you find that's what suits you best. Some babies slide naturally into routines of their own making. But don't expect a routine to be rigidly reliable all the time. Many babies have a few days now and then of extra feeding; it's thought to be due to the fact that they need extra milk because their bodies are going through a 'growth spurt' (see *breastfeeding*).

DENTAL CHECKS Dental check-ups and treatment are free while you're pregnant and for a year after your baby is born (see *teeth in pregnancy*).

DEVELOPMENT OF FETUS The major development of the unborn baby takes place in the first three months of pregnancy. During that time, most of the organs are formed and the fetus needs the extra time left mainly to

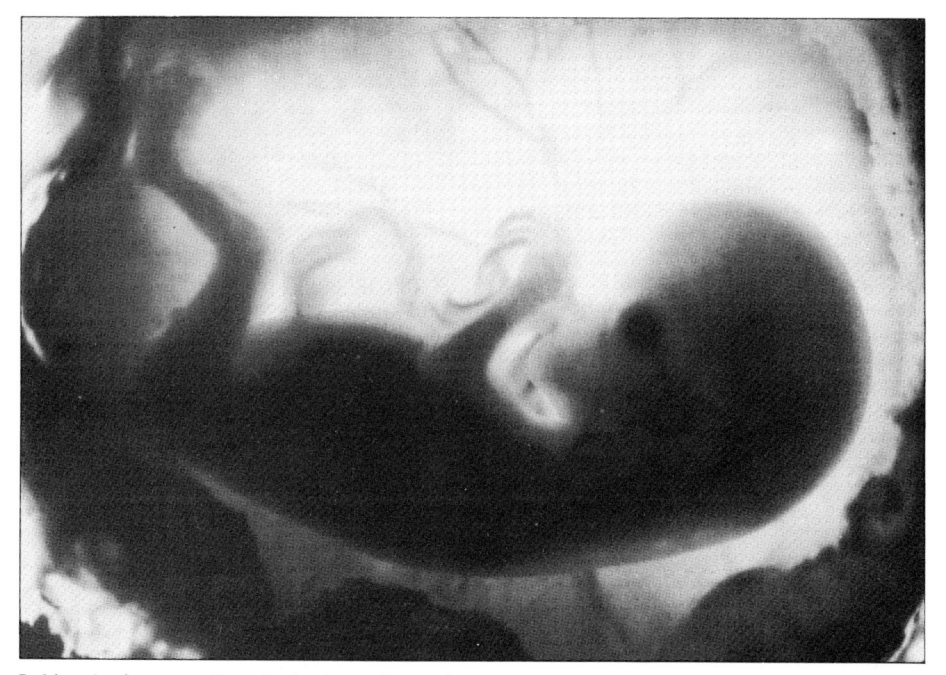

By 14 weeks of pregnancy the major development is complete.

DIABETES

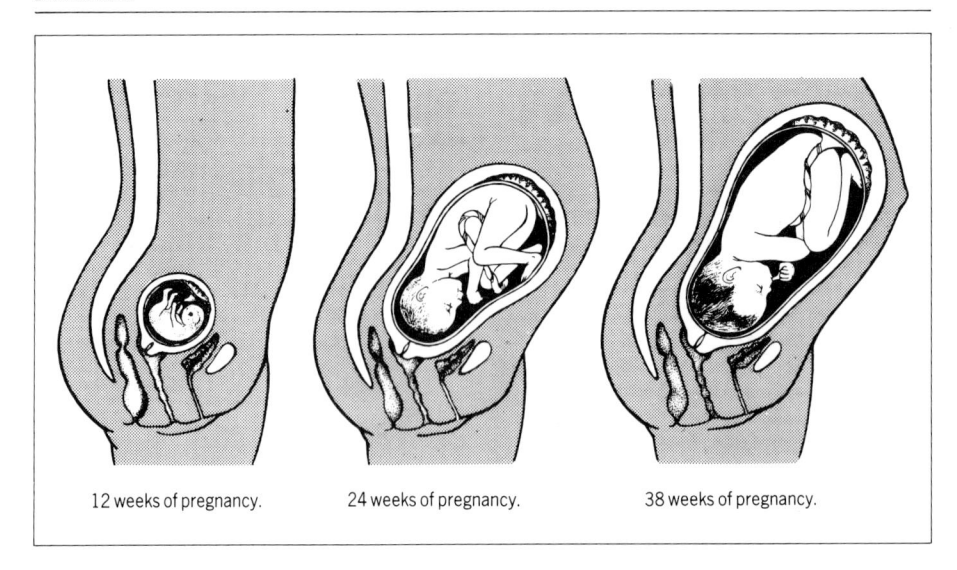

12 weeks of pregnancy.   24 weeks of pregnancy.   38 weeks of pregnancy.

mature and to grow in size. The question of when life begins is a moral and philosophical one, rather than a scientific one, as a 'potential' human being certainly exists at fertilisation when the sperm fuses with the egg. After fertilisation the egg divides again and again from two to four to eight to sixteen cells and so on, to form the *blastocyst*; within three or four days it has travelled along the *fallopian tube* (where fertilisation took place) to reach the uterus. It embeds itself in the uterine wall and by the time your period is due, the embryo is about 1 centimetre (less than half an inch) in size. During the second month of pregnancy, there is the beginning of blood circulation, and there is a heart beat. The major internal organs begin their development.

By 12 weeks, the fetus is 10 centimetres (about 4 inches) long, and the arms, legs, fingers and toes are clearly evident. The sex of the fetus would now be obvious if you could see. By 17 weeks the fetus has developed downy hair (called *lanugo*) over all his body and his eyebrows and eyelashes start to grow. By 24 weeks, his muscle development has increased, and you will be aware of fairly active movement. He measures about 30 centimetres (12 inches) from top to toe and weighs about half a kilogram (just over a pound). At 28 weeks he weighs about half his eventual birthweight and he is still very skinny.

During the last weeks of pregnancy your baby will lay down fat deposits. His lungs don't mature until the last few weeks, however, which is why so many pre-term babies have breathing difficulties at birth and for some time after. Most babies are born between 37 and 42 weeks, and the average baby weighs between 2.5 and 4.5 kilograms (5½ pounds to 10 pounds), with most babies hovering somewhere round the 3.5 kilogram mark (7½ pounds).

DIABETES Some women develop diabetes during pregnancy, and the good news is that for many women this so-called pregnancy diabetes or gestational diabetes only happens when they are pregnant, and it disappears after childbirth. However, mothers with diabetes in pregnancy warrant extra antenatal care. Diabetes is a condition caused by a lack of the hormone insulin, which is needed by the body to convert sugar into glycogen (the form in which it is stored in the body). The result is that a diabetic's blood sugar level is high and sugar may appear in her urine. Some diabetic conditions can be controlled by diet; others need injections of insulin. There are risks to the mother and her baby if the diabetes isn't kept under control, but these risks are greatly decreased with the proper care. Babies of diabetic mothers are usually on the large side, 4.5 kilograms plus (10 pounds).

DIAPHRAGM The dome-shaped muscle that separates your chest cavity from your abdomen. Towards the end of pregnancy, your enlarged uterus will press against your diaphragm – and this can make your breathing shorter and shallower (see *lightening*).

DIAPHRAGM (CONTRACEPTIVE CAP) If you have been using a diaphragm before you became pregnant, you'll need to have it checked for fit if you want to continue with this method after the baby is born. The vagina changes in size and shape after pregnancy and birth, and you may need a different size (see *family planning*).

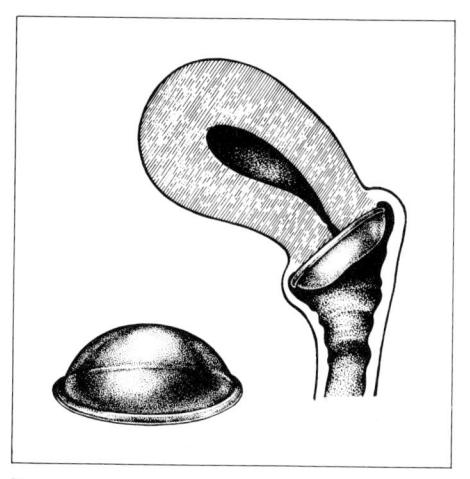

The diaphragm or contraceptive cap.

DIARRHOEA You can get the occasional bout of diarrhoea in pregnancy just as when you aren't pregnant, and there's no need to seek medical advice unless it's painful and persistent. Many women find they have a mild attack just before labour begins, which clears the bowel and rectum of fecal matter that could impede the progress of the baby's head. It also allows the intestines to rest for a while, so all the body's resources and energy can concentrate on the mammoth task of giving birth. If this happens to you, then tell the midwife, as there may be no need for an *enema* at the start of labour. Diarrhoea in new babies is rare (though more common later on, especially in bottlefed babies).

DIET Mothers who have lived on a diet of white, sliced bread and supermarket jam have gone on to have perfect babies. Some mothers are so sick in the first three months of pregnancy (and even beyond) that hardly anything they eat seems to stay down anyway; and they too have healthy babies. On the other hand, research shows that the size and health of your baby can be linked with the adequacy or otherwise of your diet. Stockbreeders have for generations acted on the premise that good health before and during pregnancy is essential for animals – but it's only now that its importance is being recognised for us humans.

In many hospitals, a dietician working with the ante-natal clinic will help you work out a healthy diet for pregnancy. There are, however, no special rules. Most of us know these days that junk food (over-refined, over-processed, artificially flavoured and coloured, loaded with preservatives and chemicals) is not good for anyone day in day out – and the same goes for you and your unborn baby. Pregnancy is a time to rethink your eating habits. If brown rice and organically grown vegetables are unavailable or unacceptable to you, you can make other changes. Make sure all the bread you eat is wholemeal, giving you valuable vitamins and other nutrients lost in the processed white variety, as well as fibre. Eat more raw food and

DILATATION

avoid the British speciality of vegetables cooked to a pulp in gallons of boiled water (which greatly reduces the vitamin content). Cut down on empty calories in cakes, biscuits and sweets. It's not just for your baby's sake that you need to eat well. A good healthy diet can help you cope with the extra physical stress of being pregnant, and ward off fatigue and sickness. If you're overweight, then it's not usually a good idea to choose pregnancy as a time to go on a reducing diet. It can sometimes be done successfully, but you need to be quite sure you aren't running the risk of going short of important nutrients, very easy to do on a slimming diet, and it matters even more when you're pregnant. Check with a diet-minded doctor if you can, or the dietician at the ante-natal clinic, whether slimming can be done safely on the diet you propose.

You can get very hungry in the days after birth, especially if you're wanting to breastfeed. The quantity and quality of hospital food is often poor, and you may need to ask friends and visitors to bring in supplements.

DILATATION The process of opening up that the *cervix* undergoes during labour. The cervix is closed throughout pregnancy and the small opening – the os – at the tip is plugged with mucus. At the end of pregnancy this mucus comes away as the *show* and shortly afterwards uterine *contractions* begin. These help to open up and draw back the cervix to allow for the descent of the baby's head. Towards the end of pregnancy, the cervix usually dilates quite painlessly, with the show still intact, and it's quite normal for an internal examination to reveal you're already 1½ or even 2 centimetres dilated (especially if you've already had a child before). The cervix needs to be 10 centimetres dilated before the process is completed, and it's at this point that the second stage of labour – the actual delivery – begins.

DILATATION AND CURETTAGE See *D & C*.

DISCHARGE It's quite normal for there to be some sort of discharge from the vagina during pregnancy, and though it doesn't have the same sort of cyclical changes you may notice when you aren't pregnant, the amount can be more profuse than you are used to. Only if it appears foul or offensive, or itchy is there any need to take medical advice (you could, for instance have *thrush*). After the baby is born you will have several days, perhaps weeks, of vaginal discharge known as *lochia*.

DISCHARGE FROM HOSPITAL See *hospital birth*.

DISPROPORTION Normally, a mother's pelvis is quite wide enough for her baby to descend head-first during labour and delivery without any problems of 'fit'. Occasionally, however, there can be disproportion, when for some reason, the size and/or shape of the pelvis won't allow a vaginal delivery. This is usually spotted ante-natally, and in late pregnancy you may be advised to have an X-ray which gives a clear picture of your baby in relation to the structure of your pelvis. This allows the obstetrician to judge whether a vaginal delivery is possible or not. If not, you will have a *caesarean section*.

Sometimes, disproportion doesn't become apparent until the mother has gone into labour. Minor degrees of disproportion don't necessarily rule out a vaginal delivery, and you may have a *trial of labour*, ending in a caesarean section only if it becomes clear that good progress isn't being made.

If disproportion is diagnosed in one pregnancy, it isn't always the case for subsequent pregnancies. You may produce a smaller baby next time round, who 'fits' you more neatly.

DIURETICS (*di-yoo-retix*) These are drugs which increase the excretion of urine – that is, they make you want to pass more water. They might be prescribed in pregnancy if you have severe fluid retention, otherwise it is best to avoid them.

DOMINO SCHEME This stands for 'domicilary-in-and-out', and it's a service involving *community midwives* that's operated with some success in different parts of the country. The idea is that you are looked after mainly by your community midwife, mostly at home, while you are pregnant. She then takes you into hospital when labour starts and, if all continues to go well, she will deliver your baby. You then go home after a few hours, with the baby and your midwife continues to look after you at home. This means that much of the first stage of labour is at home, but under the midwife, who then tells you when she thinks you should be heading for hospital, some time shortly before the start of second stage. Such a system does combine many of the advantages of home delivery with the 'insurance policy' of hospital emergency care should you need it. If you think the domino scheme would suit you, you can find out from your GP or from the community midwives in your area if the service is available locally, and whether or not you would be considered suitable for it.

DOUBLE UTERUS See *bicornuate uterus.*

DOULA *(dóoler)* This is a term recently resurrected by writers and counsellors working in the area of childbirth and post-natal care. It describes a woman – often older – found in many cultures round the world, whose specific function is to look after a new mother. She stays with her, perhaps living with her, and maybe taking over some of the usual domestic tasks, giving love, support and instruction in child care. Even in this country, the middle classes before the war often engaged a 'monthly nurse' who came and lived in for a few weeks after the birth of a new baby. These days, a new mother may have her own mother to help for a week or so, but not much more. Few employers are willing to give new fathers paternity leave. There's not a great deal of age-group mixing in modern communities, and a new mother's friends (if she has any nearby) are likely to have their own family responsibilities. Add to this the fact that there's an unspoken pressure to get back to normal as soon as possible after the birth, and perhaps we lose out. I don't think we need to go back 30 years (when my mother and her contemporaries were ordered to stay in bed for a fortnight after a confinement), but the huge upheaval that a new baby brings to your life isn't cushioned at all. It would be wonderful if every new mother could *gradually* return to a normal life without feeling self-indulgent; if she had someone to take over housework and cooking; if she had friends and family to be on 'her side'. We don't have doulas in this society but that doesn't mean we don't need practical help and friendship after childbirth. Good, mother-to-mother support is offered by organisations like the National Childbirth Trust, which has a network of post-natal support groups who can give you the chance, if you want it, of being befriended by one individual 'supporter'. Their breastfeeding counsellors give encouragement with breastfeeding. Health visitors increasingly see themselves as offering sympathetic support to new mothers, and not just advice on baby care.

If you need this sort of help, do tell someone, and ask for it. Too much unhappiness is caused by mothers soldiering on, feeling they ought to be coping marvellously, putting on a brave face yet feeling exhausted, isolated and confused (see *post-natal depression;* also Useful Addresses).

DOWN'S SYNDROME A chromosomal disorder, present from the moment of conception, affecting one baby in about 700 over all, but much more common in babies born to mothers in their late 30s and over. Down's syndrome is the most common of the mental handicaps. People with Down's syndrome (it's also known as mongolism) are mentally slower than their contemporaries, and although many can eventually learn basic skills, and to read and write, most will need care and attention throughout their lives. When a Down's baby is born, a midwife's suspicions may be aroused as there are distinctive facial characteristics, but only a doctor can make a firm diagnosis on the basis of further investigation.

The cause of Down's syndrome isn't fully understood, although older mothers (that is, mothers over 35) are more likely to give birth to Down's babies than younger mothers, so it may be something to do with the degeneration of the female egg (that doesn't explain why Down's babies can be born to mothers of any age, though). Down's syndrome can be tested for during pregnancy with *amniocentesis*. This test is usually available to women in their late 30s, or to women who have already given birth to a Down's child. If Down's syndrome is detected, the mother may be asked if she wants to consider an abortion.

DRIP   Sometimes it is necessary for a fluid (containing, for example, sugar, or a drug) to be fed gradually and directly into a person's bloodstream, rather than passing through the digestive system first as it would if it were delivered in tablet or medicine form. In these cases, a drip is set up. The fluid is allowed to drip into a vein via thin tubing ending in a needle. Labour can be induced with a drip of *oxytocin*. Sometimes a sugar drip (usually a dextrose solution) is set up in labour (see *induction; ketones*).

DRUGS   Many doctors are becoming more and more reluctant to prescribe drugs for pregnant women (apart from medication obviously needed for some long-term illness or condition). Many drugs have been used for years without any obvious effects on the unborn child, but this growing conservatism is probably wise. The thalidomide scandal of a generation ago – babies were born with varying degrees of limb deformity due to drugs their mothers took in pregnancy, prescribed for them in good faith by their doctors – shows that years can go by before harmful effects can be known.

The first three months of pregnancy are the most vulnerable for the developing fetus, and this is the time when doctors are most concerned to avoid unnecessary prescribing. On the other hand, you may develop a condition that's eminently treatable by medication (for example, *thrush* or a urine infection). As long as your doctor's aware that you're pregnant, the chances are that there is no cause for anxiety at all. Don't take non-prescription drugs bought over the counter without consulting your doctor first, but worrying whether the aspirin you took for a headache before you knew you were pregnant could spoil an otherwise enjoyable pregnancy and is just not worth it. If you are already taking drugs for some condition, check with your doctor that they are safe now that you are pregnant.

Remember, though, that smoking and alcohol are harmful. And if you're in the habit of taking other drugs – hard or soft – stop now, with medical advice and support if need be. It's well known that babies of heroin addicts are born already addicted. The same thing can happen with other opiate drugs, and even barbiturates. And valium, taken in late pregnancy, can cause convulsions in a newborn.

ECTOPIC PREGNANCY

ECLAMPSIA Nowadays this is a rare condition in pregnancy, labour or soon afterwards. The reason it's rare is mainly due to the fact that the signs of *pre-eclampsia* are almost always spotted at ante-natal checks and preventative measures taken to stop it becoming more serious. Eclampsia is characterised by convulsions and loss of consciousness. It needs emergency treatment, with drugs to stop the convulsions.

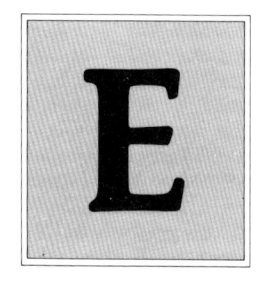

EATING IN LABOUR In most hospitals, eating during labour is not allowed. This is because if you were to require a general anaesthetic so a caesarean section could be performed you might run the risk of inhaling your stomach contents. If there was food in your stomach at the time, these contents would be acidic, and this could be dangerous for you. This risk has to be countered by the fact that a labouring woman needs to keep her strength up. If she hasn't enough carbohydrate stores in her body she will develop ketosis and this in itself is hazardous to the smooth progress of labour. Ketosis can be quickly and effectively dealt with by setting up a sugar drip, but with the inconvenience this can bring to the mother.

One school of thought says it is quite acceptable to eat and drink according to hunger and thirst in labour, because it is not right to put a routine policy into effect just in case an individual mother is one of the few who may need an emergency caesarean section. The compromise view is that certain foods and drinks are less likely to produce acid stomach contents, and these would therefore be acceptable. Speak to your consultant and ask what he thinks. It could be a sensible policy, however, to make sure you have a nutritious, easily digested meal at home, as soon as you suspect you are in labour (see *ketones*).

ECTOPIC PREGNANCY The normal site of a developing pregnancy is in the uterus. Just occasionally, the fertilised egg embeds somewhere else – usually in the *fallopian tube*, which is why ectopic pregnancy is sometimes also called tubal pregnancy. It happens because the egg is unable, for some reason, to make its way through the tube (as a result, perhaps, of some pelvic infection in the past, or perhaps an unusually long tube that has kinked). In rare cases the egg embeds in the ovary, or elsewhere. The outcome is invariably the ending of the pregnancy in one way or another, almost always within the first 10 weeks. The pregnancy may abort, and be 'lost' through the open end of the fallopian

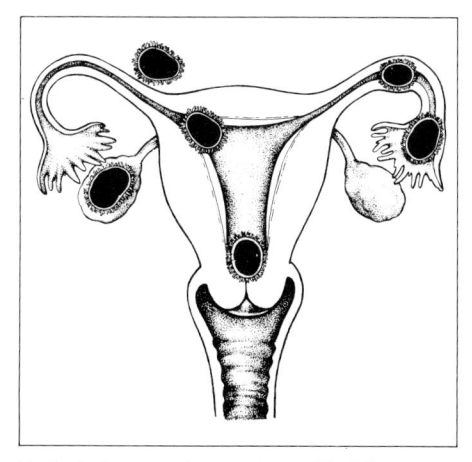

Most ectopic pregnancies occur in one of the fallopian tubes, but it is possible, though rare, for it to happen elsewhere in the sites shown.

EDD/EDC

tube, with consequent internal bleeding. There will be vaginal bleeding too. Sometimes, the fallopian tube itself may rupture. Ectopic pregnancy is serious, and it needs urgent treatment, once diagnosed, to prevent haemorrhage. The symptoms which will lead to a diagnosis are severe pain, possibly fainting and vomiting, and even collapse. In other cases, the symptoms of ectopic pregnancy are less dramatic: there may be recurrent attacks of pain, vaginal bleeding or a dark brown discharge (from the lining of the uterus). Occasionally it is necessary to remove the affected fallopian tube. Where the tube has already ruptured, there's little chance of repair, though pioneering surgical work in this area offers hope for the future. However, even if a woman has lost a fallopian tube in this way, it is still possible for her to have a subsequent normal pregnancy.

EDD/EDC You may see either or both of these sets of initial on your notes or *co-operation card*. They mean respectively estimated date of delivery/estimated date of confinement (that is, the day or approximately the day you would be expected to give birth (see *dating the pregnancy*, *length of pregnancy*).

EFFACEMENT This is the 'taking up' of the cervix, which happens at the very end of pregnancy (in a first-time mother), or together with *dilatation* during the first stage (if you've had a baby before). With effacement, the cervical canal shortens until it becomes continuous with the uterus and the vagina. It's been described in one book as being like the neck of a balloon when the balloon is blown up – the neck disappears when the balloon is fully inflated.

EMBRYO The developing baby at the start of pregnancy. Technically, the embryo becomes a fetus five weeks after conception.

EMERGENCY BIRTH Says actor Alan Alda, in the American film *Same Time Next Year* when confronted by the imminent delivery of his girlfriend's child: 'You can't have the baby here. I'm not a cab driver . . . !' Emergency births like this are unusual – and that's why you see headlines in the paper praising fathers, ambulance men, and yes, taxi drivers, as heroes of the hour. In very rare instances, a baby is born after three or four contractions in very quick succession, before the mother has realised she is in labour. Usually, the outcome is good, particularly if the baby is born at or near term. However someone – and hopefully it won't have to be the mother herself – must contact the ambulance service or the community midwife, or GP, to report what happened. Sometimes, a woman goes into strong labour and realises getting to hospital in time won't be possible. Whoever is with her needs to contact the midwife, or possibly the ambulance service again, stating clearly that the obstetric *flying squad* is needed. If the baby is born before expert help arrives, the mother needs to be made comfortable and the baby needs to be kept warm. The cutting of the cord should wait.

Emergency birth is, of course, quite different from a planned *home birth*.

EMERGENCY CAESAREAN SECTION There can be one or more of a number of reasons for this. The baby may show signs of *fetal distress*: his heart rate (and possibly other signs, too) shows he is finding being born too tiring and he is weakening; *placental abruption* where the placenta is coming away from the uterus wall; *prolapse of the umbilical cord*; when it becomes clear that there is *disproportion*, and the baby's head and your pelvis are the wrong size and shape for each other (though this is often detected ante-natally); when labour isn't progressing at what the doctor feels is a satisfactory rate (by no means a cut and dried situation; some doctors are keener to intervene with surgery than others, and feel it's safer to do so when labour is slow or erratic). Other obstetricians give 'nature' more time to take its course.

EMOTIONS AFTER THE BIRTH

Unless you already have an *epidural* anaesthetic in place, you will probably be given a general anaesthetic as it can put you under straight away with no waiting (see *caesarean section*).

EMERGENCIES IN LABOUR Any sudden bleeding in labour, and rapid deterioration in the condition of the mother, signs of severe fetal distress – all can be symptoms of an emergency situation. Pre-term labour – labour before the 37th week – is potentially less than ideal, but with newer methods of neo-natal care, the outlook for early babies is very good. Good ante-natal care these days often spots potential emergencies before they cause problems.

EMERGENCIES IN PREGNANCY
Bleeding in pregnancy is cause for concern, and sudden severe bleeding is a definite emergency, as is severe and unremitting pain. Either of these could herald a *miscarriage*, pre-term labour, *haemorrhage, ectopic pregnancy, placenta praevia* or *placental abruption*. An emergency needs the obstetric *flying squad* to deal with it and/or speedy admission into hospital. Convulsions (fits) in pregnancy can be a sign of *eclampsia*, and this too is an emergency.

EMOTIONS AFTER THE BIRTH You may feel tired, yet exhilarated, after giving birth. It's quite common to feel very high for sometime afterwards in fact, and to feel a sense of oneness with the rest of womankind, particularly if this is your first baby. It's also common to feel tearful and moody a few days after the birth but this feeling generally passes. If it doesn't pass, or if it goes away and then returns in a different form, you should seek advice. Post-natal depression has many manifestations and symptoms, but it can

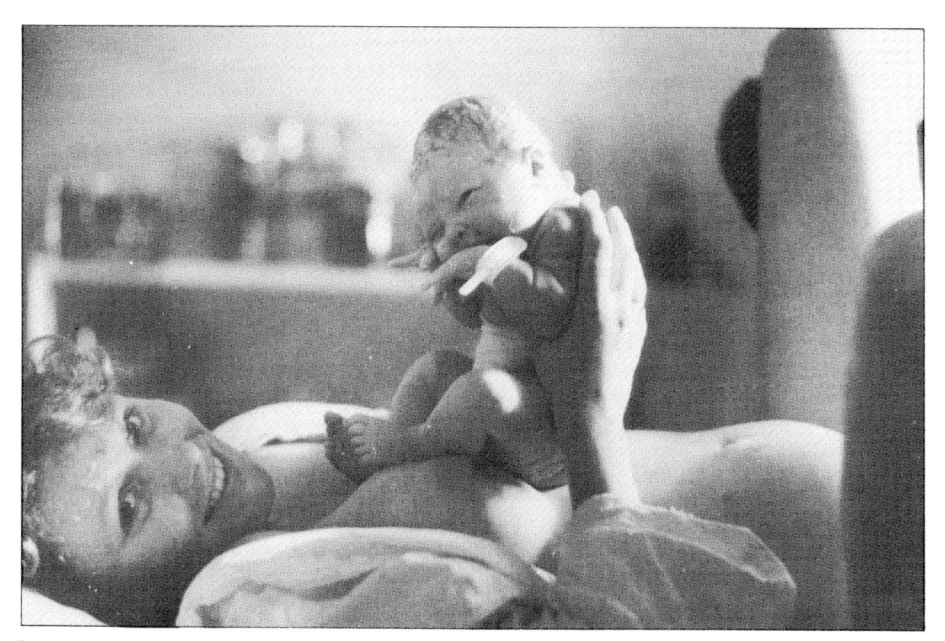

Emotions vary but are often described as ones of joy, tenderness, pride and elation.

always be helped with the right approach and treatment. On the positive side, lots of mothers have what I have heard termed 'post-natal elation'! Pregnancy, birth, feeding and caring become all part of a happy, whole experience, and whereas the tensions and difficulties of being a new mother are there too, they never come anywhere near theatening the overwhelming joy of it all (see *post-natal blues, post-natal depression*).

EMOTIONS DURING PREGNANCY At the beginning, and at the end of pregnancy, many women say they feel their emotions fluctuating (though this can happen all the way through, too!). Maybe it's 'your hormones' as they say, or perhaps its the realisation of the impending changes to your lifestyle that your baby will bring you, and the acceptance of the huge responsibility. Towards the end, sheer impatience with waiting, and tiredness can make you irritable and edgy. Relaxation therapy – taught at ante-natal classes – could help you. Share your feelings with other women and with your partner, and speak to your doctor or midwife if you find your emotions are a problem to you, or if you find you are becoming very anxious (see *anxiety in pregnancy*).

ENDOMETRIUM The mucus membrane which forms the inner lining of the uterus. After conception, this membrane thickens and the blood vessels it is supplied by increase in size ready for implantation of the embryo. The endometrium is called the decidua during pregnancy; after delivery it is gradually shed.

ENEMA The midwife may give you an enema as part of the '*prepping*' procedure when you're admitted to hospital in early labour. You'll be asked to lie on your side and she will insert the contents of a small bag of salted water into your back passage. The result is that you will have the urge to empty your bowels, which rids the rectum (back passage) of any faeces. The advantage of having an empty rectum and lower bowel in labour is that no hard impacted faeces can prevent or delay the descent of the baby's head down the birth canal (remember the rectum is just next door to the vagina). The other advantage – if advantage it is – is that there is supposed to be less risk of faeces being pushed out with the birth of the baby, which may be embarrassing to you if you are sensitive in that respect. The disadvantage of an enema is that it is rather an uncomfortable procedure; the action of having your rectum stimulated in this way can be very unpleasant to many women, and the whole notion of being given an enema can be distressing. Uterine contractions can be stronger after an enema, as the contractions of the lower bowel seem to trigger off a sympathetic action.

If you are really constipated, then an enema can be a good idea. If you're not, and especially if you have recently opened your bowels, then the advantage of an enema isn't clear. Tell the midwife if you have just been to the lavatory (in the last few hours), and if she still feels you'd be better off with an enema, ask if suppositories couldn't be used instead – their action is slower and less strong than an enema (see *constipation*).

ENERGY SPURT A very common phenomenon later in pregnancy, often coinciding with the start of labour. You might feel like papering a room, baking a dozen loaves of bread or scrubbing the kitchen floor. Could it be your body putting you on a physical 'high' in preparation for labour?

ENGAGEMENT OF HEAD Most babies are born head first, and they engage in the pelvis before this happens. This means that the head drops right down, and the widest part of the head is actually through the pelvic brim. The midwife can usually feel quite easily whether the head is engaged or not. In a first pregnancy, the head engages at about the 37th week. In a second or subsequent pregnancy the head might not engage until just before labour; some women of African descent may find their babies' heads don't engage until later either. Later engagement in these cases simply reflects a slight difference in the shape of the pelvic bones. It's a good sign for a straightforward labour once the head is engaged. If the head doesn't engage, it could mean (among other things) that the baby is *occipito posterior* or that the placenta is in the way (see *placenta praevia*).

ENGORGEMENT OF BREASTS This is a rather uncomfortable – yet temporary – condition that quite commonly happens during the first week or so of breastfeeding (though it can happen at any time thereafter, as well, under certain conditions). It's caused by the great increase in blood supply to the breasts, together with the effect of the milk 'coming in' on the second, third or fourth day after delivery. The breasts are full, hard, tense and hot. The best way to avoid engorgement is to feed your baby frequently (not always easy if you have a sleepy baby) and to offer your baby a feed as soon as you feel your breasts are becoming uncomfortable. If the engorgement means your breasts are hard and the nipple difficult for your baby to latch on to, try to soften the breasts by gently expressing a little milk before a feed. There are a number of ways of dealing with engorgement, which almost always cures itself with extra feeding, and a midwife or breastfeeding counsellor will be able to offer suggestions.

If you don't wish to breastfeed, you will still experience engorgement as your breasts will initially fill with milk. The traditional and usually effective way of relieving discomfort and hastening the disappearance of the milk is to wear a tight uplifting bra, which binds you very closely, and to restrict your fluid intake. Hormone drugs can be prescribed by the doctor, though this is done less often these days, and usually only in cases where the baby has died (see *latching on*).

ENTONOX The brand name given to the mixture of 50 per cent nitrous oxide and 50 per cent oxygen ('gas and air' is its popular though incorrect name), commonly used as a pain-relieving drug during labour and delivery. It's contained in a cylinder, attached to some tubing which ends in a face mask. You place the mask over your nose and mouth and breathe in to get a dose. It's simple to use, and doesn't have a build-up effect in your body. It's always self-administered, so when you've had enough of it, the hand holding the mask simply falls away and you can't breathe it in any more. The typical effect is to feel woozy or drunk (though not happy-drunk) for a few seconds at a time. You need to breathe it in at the start of a contraction, so the effect is at its height at the peak of the same contraction. Some mothers find it's a very acceptable form of relief. It doesn't have the disadvantage of leaving the baby sleepy at birth, and you only use as much as you feel you need. However, with a very difficult or painful labour the effects of Entonox aren't very strong, and some women really dislike the sensation of having a rubber thing over their face (memories of the dentist's chair, perhaps). Others hate the feeling – albeit temporary – of being slightly-out-of-control and 'not all there'. If you get a chance to practise with Entonox (at an ante-natal class or clinic), take it, so you have some chance of knowing what your reaction might be in advance.

EPIDURAL ANAESTHESIA The epidural space lies between the bony column of your spine and the spinal cord itself, which is full of vital nerve fibres. Among these nerve fibres are sensory fibres, which carry sensations to the brain. By injecting an anaesthetic into the epidural space, the sensory nerve fibres from the uterus can be numbed, and the sensation of pain during labour is wiped out, while leaving the mother fully conscious. The epidural needs to be administered by an anaesthetist, who inserts a very thin needle into the mother's back, having numbed the area of insertion with local anaesthetic first, and from there the needle is inserted into the

EPIDURAL ANAESTHESIA

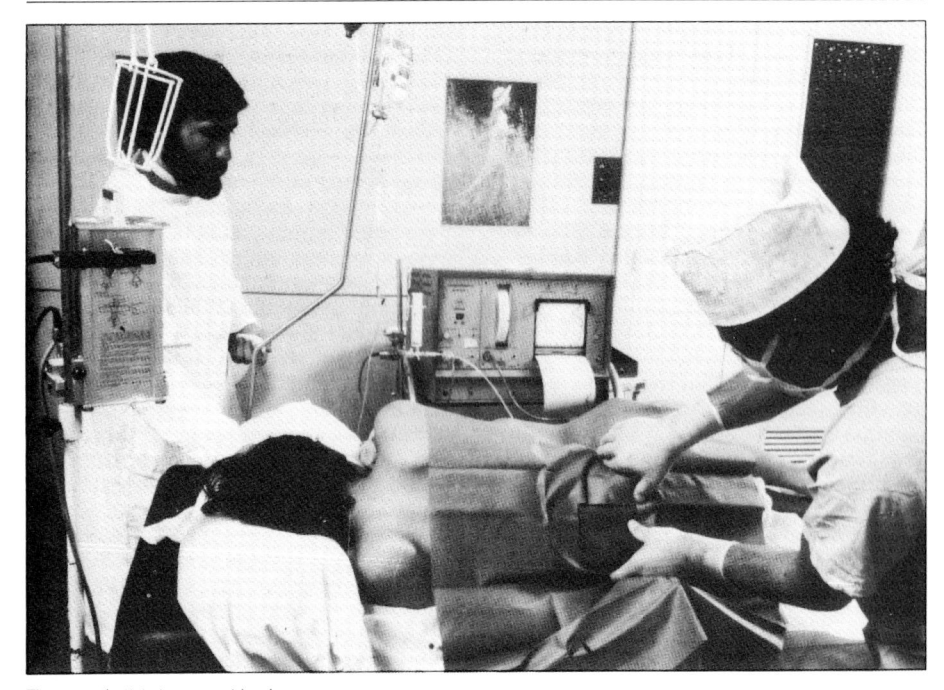

The anaesthetist gives an epidural.

epidural space. A fine catheter (tubing) then goes through the needle and the needle is withdrawn, leaving the catheter in place. The anaesthetic can go into the epidural space through the catheter, and top-ups can be added, when needed. The catheter is fixed to your back with sticky tape. It takes about 10 or 15 minutes to administer the epidural and it starts to work shortly after that.

There are various points to consider if you feel you might be interested in opting for an epidural. The trade-off for lack of pain could be a great increase in the medical management of your baby's birth. You will need to be monitored throughout (that is, a machine is attached to you that measures the strength of your contractions) and your baby will also be monitored with a *fetal monitor*. You may well have a drip to speed up your labour, and statistics show you have a greater chance of having a forceps delivery (partly because you don't have the sensation of wanting to *bear down*). You may need a catheter to pass urine, as you won't be able to feel the usual sensations of opening your bladder. The epidural can cause a drop in blood pressure, and so your blood pressure will be taken at frequent intervals to keep a check on this. You won't be able to change your position much (you couldn't walk, anyway, because your legs will be numb). Epidurals don't always work perfectly; they sometimes have an effect down one side only, leaving all the pain on the other. Other possible after-effects are a long-lasting headache and very rarely numbness in the legs – and, even more rarely, thankfully, paralysis. All these risks are considerably reduced when the epidural is given by an anaesthetist skilled and well-practised in giving them. Epidural anaesthesia has a much less obvious effect on the baby than other pain relieving drugs like *pethidine*, but even so, small amounts of the anaesthetic do get into the baby's system, with no apparent long-term effect, however.

The advantages for you may well outweigh the disadvantages, and increased management, for instance, may be a small price to pay for the chance of pain-free labour. You may find yourself starting off labour easily and well, and wish to keep the option of an epidural in reserve, rather than having one right from the start. If you wish to be certain of having an epidural at any time, then ask if this will be possible in advance. Most large maternity units will have the facility; some smaller ones don't, because they can't rely on having an anaesthetist available. If you know you are to have a *caesarean section*, it may be possible for this to be done with an epidural rather than a general anaesthetic, and this could be better for the baby and you, as well as giving you the chance to be conscious during the birth. An epidural is sometimes recommended for a breech birth; the reason is that the epidural takes away the urge to push. This can be an advantage as a breech can give you the urge to push too soon, before the cervix is fully dilated. Some doctors recommend an epidural in labour where the mother has high blood pressure, as the blood pressure lowering effect of the epidural can be beneficial.

For some women, an epidural is simply not an attractive proposition. They prefer to be involved and in control of their labour, rather than start off the chain of medical intervention that the epidural may mean. For others, however, the prospect of epidural anaesthesia quite simply removes any anxiety about labour and birth.

EPISIOTOMY This is a cut, made by the midwife or doctor, in the perineum (the skin between the vagina and the anus) just before the baby is born. The reasons given for an episiotomy are to help the baby be born more quickly (as it enlarges the exit for the baby and in the case of a pre-term baby this protects his skull); to avoid a tear in the perineum; to allow a forceps delivery; to help a baby out who's in an awkward position (for instance, a breech); to avoid the mother having to push for too long (which is thought by some to predispose to a prolapse of the uterus later on). In general an episiotomy is made when the perineum is stretched and taut, so you shouldn't feel it, although many midwives give a shot of anaesthetic anyway. After the birth, you will be sutured (sewn up). Over the following days the stitches will gradually dissolve and your perineum will heal.

There has been a lot of controversy in recent years about episiotomy. It's become clear that in many hospitals episiotomies are made more or less as routine, and that one midwife's or doctor's feelings about whether cutting is necessary may be different from another's. Of course, there are situations where an episiotomy can be life-saving – a baby in distress needs to be born soon, and an episiotomy could save vital minutes. What has started to concern people, however, is the way episiotomy can lead to problems, days, weeks even months after the baby has been born, and these problems are mainly to do with the stitching up afterwards. Even shortly after the birth, a woman who is kept waiting hours to be stitched (it can happen on a busy maternity unit) is uncomfortable, and impatient to leave the delivery room. Stitching up should never be painful or uncomfortable, by the way, and if you feel the slightest little pinprick, ask for more anaesthetic.

The quality of stitching varies greatly. Some women have found that they have needed to be restitched as the stitching has broken down. Stitching that's too tight causes the vaginal opening to be smaller, leading to distressing sexual problems later on. Almost all women who have had an episiotomy find that sitting down can be painful – if you're unlucky, excruciating – for the next few days, whatever the standard of your stitching up. Once you have had an episiotomy with one birth, your chances of another one next time are increased, as scar tissue is not as elastic as it could be, and your perineum may not stretch very well when your next baby is being born. Of course, most women end up

EQUIPMENT FOR BABY

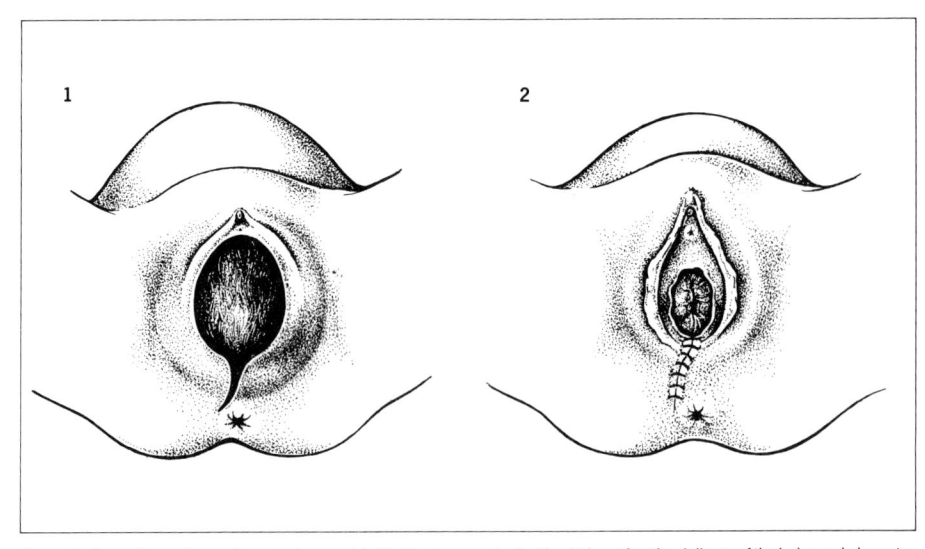

The cut in the perineum is usually made to one side (1). It is then repaired with stitches after the delivery of the baby and placenta (2).

regarding episiotomy as a minor inconvenience, and any problems associated with it soon fade, but a sufficiently large number of others report difficulties that have given rise to a re-think among many midwives and doctors, and in some units, routine episiotomies are less common than previously. Newer research suggests that small tears can heal better than episiotomies, and that an upright position in second stage can help the perineum to stretch better. Exercising your perineum (by doing *pelvic floor exercises* throughout pregnancy) may help, as can massaging your perineum with a bland oil to make the tissues more supple. However, the controversy continues as to whether episiotomies should be regarded as 'last resort' intervention only. Some midwives and obstetricians feel that the reason prolapse of the uterus is now so very uncommon is at least partly due to the great increase in the episiotomy rate in the last fifteen years or so. There's no doubt that prolonged and strained pushing in second stage, particularly while the mother is lying down, can have a weakening effect on the muscles supporting the uterus. Whether this weakening can be avoided by episiotemy is questionable, to say the least. Given that the risks and problems resulting from cutting and stitching are now well-documented, there can no longer be any justification for routine episiotomy.

EQUIPMENT FOR BABY Towards the end of pregnancy, you'll be wanting to prepare your home and your life for the new baby. This includes working out what the baby's practical needs will be; though you really don't need to get many things before she's born, you'll have less chance to go shopping afterwards. Remember almost anything can be bought second-hand if you are watchful for safety pointers. My own local paper always has at least six advertisements every night for prams, almost invariably in 'v.g.c.', for example. The only thing you really should buy new is a cot mattress, for reasons of hygiene.

Of course, it's nice to buy everything new if you want to and can afford it, and certain items are more difficult to find in a good second-hand condition.

EXERCISE IN PREGNANCY

Here's a very basic list for the items your baby will need in the first month of life.

Somewhere to sleep – cot, crib or pram
Bedding for the above – several sheets plus warm, washable covers, but no pillow
Some means of transport for trips outdoors – pram or fully reclinable pushchair or baby sling
Bedding for above – same as cot/crib folded over. A cover-all pouch for the baby sling is a good idea in winter
Something for bathing – a baby bath, or a washing up bowl will do at first.
Feeding equipment if you don't intend to breastfeed – at least four bottles and teats, plus a large plastic container for sterilising unit and fluid or tablets
Nappies – either towelling or disposable or both; plus nappy buckets, plastic pants and nappy pins
Toiletries – baby soap, lotion or cream, flannels and towels, cotton wool
Clothing – stretch suits (babygros), vests, cardigans, shawls, hats
Restraint for car – the only safe ways for a new baby to travel in a car are in a carrycot with a restraint fixed correctly in the car, or in a special seat designed for a young infant.

In addition to this, a changing mat is useful, as is a bouncing cradle (a framed chair, made of fabric – handy for a small baby to be parked in when awake) (see *bathing, bedding, clothes for baby, nappies*).

EXERCISE IN PREGNANCY Keeping fit and healthy in pregnancy is one of the best ways to prepare yourself for labour and birth. A suitable amount of exercise is therefore a good idea as part of this. Don't start any vigorous exercise in pregnancy (your body won't be used to it), but if you normally jog, swim energetically, play tennis or whatever, and your doctor approves, don't let pregnancy put you off. The only really hazardous forms of exercise are the sort where you run the risk of falling or being injured, so you'd be wise to avoid horse racing, judo or mountain climbing. After mid-pregnancy you'll probably not want to engage in strenuous exercise, so that will rule out aerobics or tennis, but swimming is an excellent exercise you can do all the way through, and of course you control the energy output yourself. Yoga is also good exercise, as long as you stick to positions that are suitable for pregnancy (ask your teacher), and it can increase your

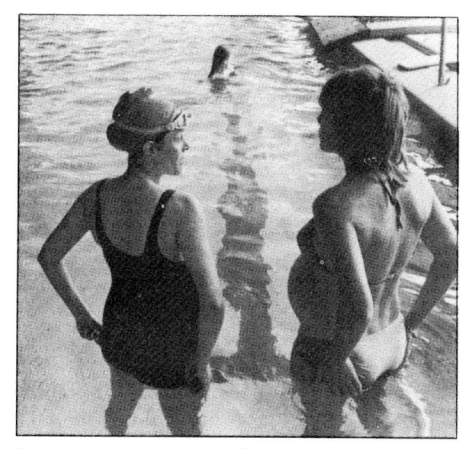

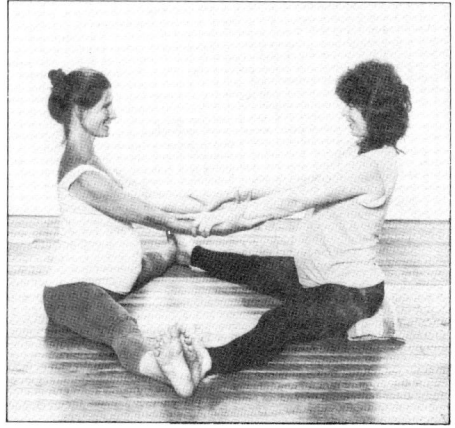

Swimming and yoga are useful forms of exercise during pregnancy.

EXPRESSING MILK

suppleness and flexibility. *Pelvic floor exercises* are simple, and help to prepare the perineum and the pelvic muscles for childbirth. Many ante-natal classes teach exercises, and there are some good books on the subject.

EXPRESSING MILK You will probably not need to do this in the normal course of events. If, however, your baby is separated from you for any reason (perhaps because he is ill), you will need to express milk to stimulate your breasts to get milk production underway. He can have the milk later by bottle or tube. You can express with an electric *breast pump*, or use a hand pump, or you can express by hand. A midwife, health visitor or breastfeeding counsellor will give you advice on expressing and will help you choose the right sort of pump for your needs. Some mothers find it handy to be able to express milk in order to be able to leave it for someone else to give while they go out for a while (you need to express it and then store it in a container that you've properly sterilised, and then you keep the milk covered in the fridge for up to 24 hours. It can also be deep frozen for up to six months).

Babies with some sort of defect (like a *cleft palate*) which prevents normal sucking can be given expressed breast milk by bottle. Gentle expressing in cases of *engorgement* can sometimes help to soften the breast and nipple in order to help the baby feed.

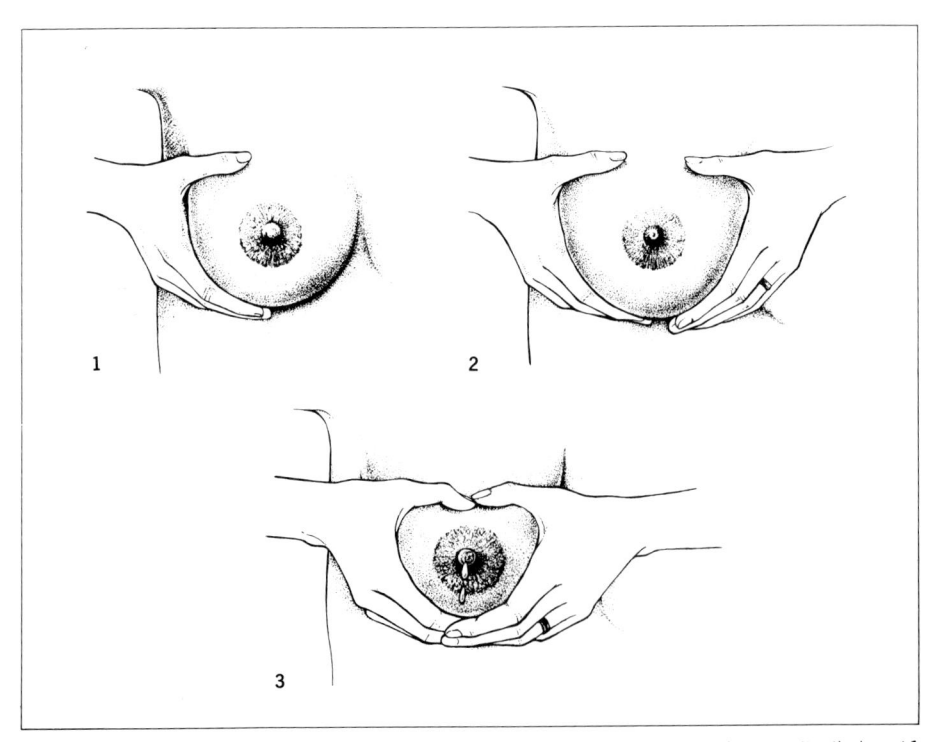

This is one method of hand-expressing which many women find comfortable and effective. Begin by supporting the breast **1** and using the thumbs to give very gentle and even massage towards the areola **2**. Gentle pressure on the milk reservoirs behind the areola will cause milk to come out through the nipple.

days later the fertilised ovum reaches the uterus and it embeds in the uterine lining. If it stays in the fallopian tube, the pregnancy is *ectopic*.

FALSE LABOUR   This isn't at all uncommon, and midwives are quite used to admitting women who are sure they are in labour, and yet whose contractions soon cease. In the days or weeks leading up to your delivery date, you may feel the *Braxton-Hicks contractions* getting more obvious, and it's easy to confuse these with the longer, more regular contractions of true labour.

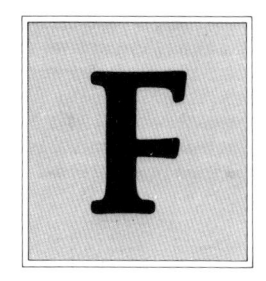

FACE PRESENTATION   Usually an unborn baby near the end of pregnancy has his head pointing downwards, his face towards your backbone and his head well-flexed, that is, with his chin tucked in. This gives the best and smoothest way to be born. Occasionally, however, a baby may have his head flexed backwards; his chin points upwards instead of inwards. The result is that instead of the top of his head being the first part to be born, his face is what comes out first. Problems with labour and birth are by no means inevitable with a face presentation, but progress is likely to be slower than normal. If the baby is in a posterior position, as well as presenting by the face – that is if he is facing towards your front – there is a possibility he could get stuck if he doesn't turn spontaneously. To avoid this possibility, the doctor may decide to use *forceps* to rotate the baby and help him out, and in fact about half of all face presentations end up being delivered by *caesarean section*. After a face presentation, the baby often looks a bit bruised and battered, but this all disappears without a trace.

FALLOPIAN TUBES   These are two narrow canals that lead from the uterus at one end to the ovary at the other. They are each about 4 inches long. When the egg is released from the ovary at ovulation, it is wafted along the fallopian tube, and if fertilisation takes place, it happens within the tube itself. About five

FALSE PREGNANCY   A woman who really wants to become pregnant may actually show some of the signs of pregnancy – growing abdomen, breast changes and even an absence of periods – yet a pregnancy test proves negative. Vaginal or abdominal examination shows nothing, either. False pregnancy like this demonstrates the power the emotions can sometimes have over the body.

FAMILY DOCTOR   See *GP*

FAMILY MEDICAL HISTORY   The background to your family's health will be asked about at your *booking appointment* at the hospital ante-natal clinic. This is to check whether you or your family have certain inheritable medical conditions that could affect the outcome of your pregnancy. For example, you'll be asked if there are twins in your family, and whether there is anybody with diabetes.

FAMILY PLANNING   Unless you truly don't mind when you become pregnant again, you'll need to consider some form of contraception fairly soon after the birth of your baby, though women vary in how quickly they feel ready to have sexual intercourse again, and you should not rush yourself if you feel too tired or too sore. If you're fully breastfeeding, you'll have some form of 'natural' protection, as breastfeeding can keep levels of the hormone prolactin, which prevents *ovulation*, high. But it's unwise to rely on this: you can ovulate without knowing (as it can happen without menstruation having started) and it's also been shown that prolactin levels can fall when breastfeeds become less frequent. Unless you are breastfeeding very frequently, round the clock (as we tend not to do in this country), you can't guarantee any contraceptive protection from breastfeeding. However most women find that breastfeeding delays the return of menstruation, and some find their periods don't return until breastfeeding ceases altogether.

If you decide you want to use some other more reliable method of contraception, you may want to think about a change to another sort after the baby's born. Barrier methods – such as the sheath – may suit you. If you want to use a *diaphragm* (cap) you'll need to have one fitted at the family planning clinic or by your doctor, and if you've used one before, you should see your doctor because you may need a different size. In recent years, the coil (IUD) has been reassessed, and some experts no longer recommend it for women who have not yet completed their families because of the risks of pelvic infections and ectopic pregnancy.

The Pill can be prescribed even if you are breastfeeding, though you'll be advised to choose the progestogen-only mini-pill as the combined pill (oestrogen and progesterone) may possibly suppress the milk supply. Nevertheless, you won't be alone if you feel you'd prefer to avoid all drugs (including the Pill) while you're breastfeeding. Minute amounts of hormone from both sorts of Pill do reach the breast milk, and whereas standard medical opinion in this country assumes this is not harmful in any way, some mothers simply prefer to choose another method. There is a good argument in favour of avoiding the Pill until you're quite sure breastfeeding is established, as giving your body the chance to build up a good supply could in theory at least be affected by the hormone in the Pill.

Natural methods of contraception – watching for temperature changes and vaginal mucus changes – can be used while breastfeeding, though symptoms may be irregular. You need a high degree of commitment and knowledge for these methods to work, but if you have these qualities, plus luck, then natural methods may well be the method that suits you.

FATHERS It's a shame to appear to reduce fathers to one single entry in this book. Most of the book has been written with the knowledge that the majority of babies arrive to two parents who have some degree of commitment to each other, and in the hope that most fathers will want to share in the happiness and responsibility pregnancy and childbirth bring. These days, fathers are usually present when their babies are born, and most find it a positive experience; some even find it gives them the chance to get in touch with depths of feelings and emotions they didn't realise they possessed! If you really don't want to be there, then no one should make you feel you have to, but it's worth considering whether your partner would feel happier with someone who loves and supports her giving her gentle encouragement. Going to ante-natal classes together can give you both some idea of what's going to happen, and help you learn how you can work together to make for a happier birth. However, no mother should feel she has to have her man there. Labour and birth may go better if she can relate directly to the midwife, without her relationship with her partner taking precedence. This is something to be decided by the couple – together.

After the birth take every chance to cuddle and hold your newborn baby. Some men feel awkward with tiny babies, and some women do too, but you'll both soon get used to it. It's becoming recognised these days that fathers also need support after the birth in their new role, and in one or two places fathers' support groups have been set up.

FATHERS

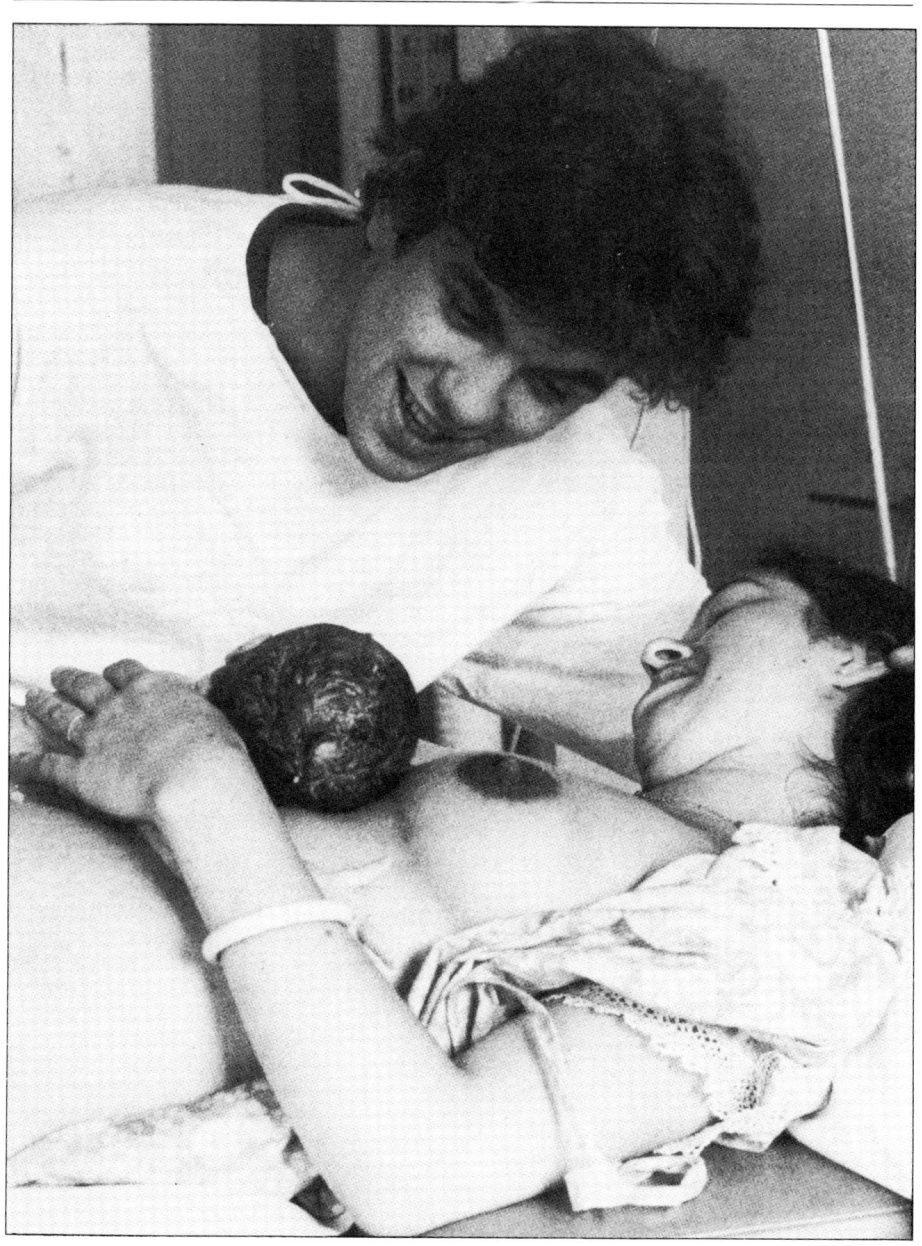

Birth is an exciting time for fathers too, and one which many want to share.

59

FEAR OF CHILDBIRTH

FEAR OF CHILDBIRTH Something that's generally less of a problem, now that the risks of childbirth are so minimal compared with years ago. It's been said that being afraid of birth can increase the tension and anxiety you feel in labour and this makes labour longer and more painful as a result. Much of today's ante-natal teaching aims to resolve any residual fears and anxieties by helping you to understand labour and birth, and giving you confidence in your ability to give birth safely and to cope with painful contractions. Women whose fear is great enough to prevent them wanting to conceive, however much they want children, or whose pregnancy is marred by fear, can be helped by skilled counselling (perhaps from a sympathetic doctor or midwife) or simply by being able to talk over their fears with their partner or with other women.

FEEDING There's no argument that *breastfeeding* gives the healthiest possible start to a baby's life, but of course there is a choice. *Bottle feeding* with modern formula milk is a substitute for breastfeeding and it is used when breastfeeding isn't possible for some reason, or when the mother doesn't wish to breastfeed. The majority of bottle fed babies grow and develop well, though health problems in the first year are far commoner in bottle fed babies, and there is evidence that allergy and later health problems are linked with bottle feeding. Although breastfeeding is on the increase, and babies in the UK are being breastfed for longer, there will always be a need for high quality baby milk, and a mother's right to choose *is* important. If the thought or the reality of breastfeeding makes you unhappy, choose the bottle – remembering that problems with breastfeeding can usually be solved with the right sort of advice. If you're neutral about feeding, with no strong preferences either way, then it can be a good idea to give breastfeeding a try. Even if you decide to bottle feed in the end, even one week, one day, or even one feed of breast milk has been shown to give some measurable protection against illness in infancy. It's also easier to switch from breast to bottle than the other way round.

FERTILISATION See *conception*.

FETAL DISTRESS A term used to describe the condition of the fetus during labour, when there are signs present that the fetus runs the risk of having insufficient oxygen. A long, tiring or difficult labour can predispose to fetal distress, as can severe *pre-eclampsia*. Light-for-dates and premature babies are also more likely to suffer distress. The signs that the midwife or doctor will watch for are a marked increase or decrease in the fetal heart rate, and meconium (the bowel motion of the fetus) in the amniotic fluid. There are varying degrees of fetal distress, and in some cases there may be mild signs that are just temporary – the fetus simply recovers. In severe cases, however, the obstetrician will want to be sure the baby is born sooner rather than later. This might mean an *emergency caesarean section*, *episiotomy* and/or *forceps*.

FETAL MONITOR A machine used during labour to record the strength of your contractions and the heart rate of your baby. A heart rate showing a consistent drop, or worrying irregularities can indicate the baby is distressed, and needs to be born soon to avoid risking his health or even his life. The type of monitor in widest use today is a machine attached to an electrode in a wire clip that fastens to the baby's scalp. The machine records the baby's heart rate on a small screen, and there may be a paper print-out as well. Your contractions are recorded by means of a sensor strapped to your abdomen and in fact some monitors use a small ultrasound detector which is also strapped to your tummy, to pick up the heart rate, instead of a scalp electrode.

The traditional way of monitoring a baby's heart is for the doctor or midwife to listen to it, by placing a stethoscope or ear trumpet on the mother's abdomen at regular intervals throughout labour. The fetal monitor gives a continuous picture of the heart rate, and, though this should have advantages, the benefits of continuous fetal monitoring are by no means unquestionable. Firstly, the mother is usually forced to be confined to bed while she is being monitored (unless she has one of the newer telemetry machines which allow her to walk about) and this in itself may slow up labour, and, some suspect, cause fetal distress. Secondly, the insertion of the scalp electrode must surely be felt as painful by the baby (common sense indicates this, though there's no evidence that there are long-term effects). There are also occasional incidents of misplacing the electrode where the baby is not presenting by the top of the head. Thirdly, the machines, like all machines, are not always reliable. This means there must be a slight risk that they register distress where none is present, which leads to caesarean deliveries and forceps deliveries which may not have been necessary. And the converse must be true, as well, with the possibility that real fetal distress is not registered. There is a feeling among some midwives and mothers that fetal monitoring can distract from other clinical signs of fetal distress, which distances the mother from the people looking after her. However, there is no doubt that many women feel reassured by watching their baby's heart rate in this way.

At the end of a problem pregnancy, or where there's some reason to suspect the baby may be at risk, short periods of monitoring every so often can help the doctor assess the condition of the baby, and the reasonably accurate picture this should give can be very reassuring, too.

The clinical benefits of routine fetal monitoring – of monitoring virtually all labours, and particularly first ones – haven't been demonstrated. The 'moderate' view – at the moment – seems to be that monitoring can be helpful to mothers who have been judged 'high risk', or who are anxious for one reason or another, but it is not necessary for others, and won't be until the advantages are shown to outweigh the disadvantages.

FETAL MOVEMENTS You will probably start to notice your baby moving in the fifth month of pregnancy. It's called *quickening* and thereafter you'll find he gets more vigorous and active – often when you're wanting to get some sleep! The last few weeks may show less movement, simply because there's less room in the uterus for physical jerks. Nevertheless, if you notice no movement at all for 24 hours or more, contact your ante-natal clinic. The chances are that there's nothing to worry about, and the clinic will soon be able to confirm this by checking the baby's heart beat. But because lack of movement is one of the first signs of a baby in distress, checking is a wise precaution. Some clinics issue *kick charts* to mothers whose pregnancies need to be watched especially closely.

FETUS Technically, the unborn baby is an *embryo* until the end of the seventh week after fertilisation. It is then termed a fetus.

FIBRE IN DIET Fibre is the key nutritional catchword of the 70s and 80s. It used to be called 'roughage' – and it refers to the cell walls of plants and cereals. Fibre provides your diet with bulk which helps keep your bowels in good working order and so avoiding any tendency to *constipation*, a common complaint in pregnancy. Fibre is present in wholegrains, fresh fruit and vegetables.

FIRST FEED If both you and the baby are well after delivery, you can offer the first breastfeed straight away. The sucking will stimulate a hormonal action that causes the uterus to contract and so expel the placenta (although where routine injections are made to stimulate this, this particular advantage is somewhat overridden); you can enjoy the closeness and contact with your baby, and

FIRST STAGE OF LABOUR

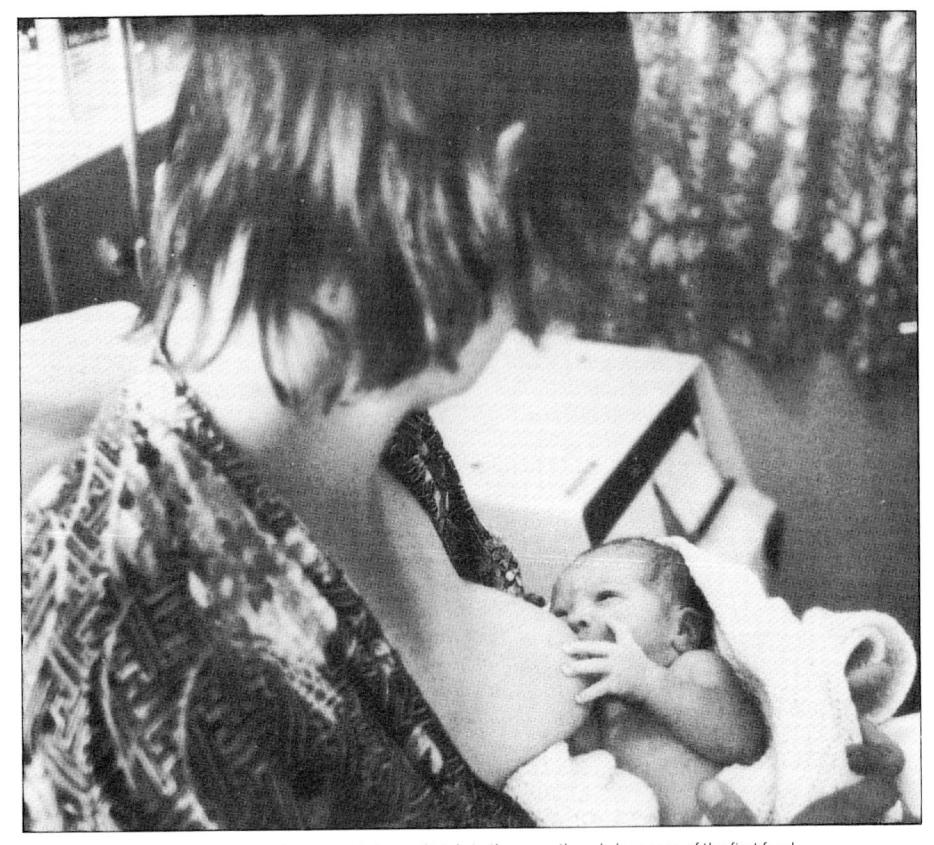

This baby is only minutes old – yet she responds immediately to the warmth and closeness of the first feed.

because she will be particularly alert at this stage (if you have avoided drugs) she will enjoy looking at you. She will get some of your valuable *colostrum* too. Some babies don't actually suck at this point but giving them the chance to see you, smell you and taste you is worth it. If you don't want to breastfeed, the first bottle feed could be given at this time too.

FIRST STAGE OF LABOUR Labour is divided into three stages. The first stage is usually the longest. It encompasses all of labour up to the point of full *dilatation* when the cervix is fully open and taken up, and the baby's head is right down ready to make progress through the birth canal. Throughout the first stage, the uterus contracts and, typically, the contractions gradually get longer, more frequent and stronger (see *labour, second stage of labour, third stage of labour*).

FLAT BABIES A term used to describe babies who appear to have problems with breathing at birth. It's not very scientific or even very descriptive as a term and doctors tend to avoid it.

FLAT NIPPLES Nipples come in lots of shapes and sizes. One variation is the 'flat' nipple that doesn't stand out very much, though with stimulation it usually does a little. The potential problem with flat nipples is that there is less for the baby to latch on to when feeding, which makes good positioning difficult to achieve without a little more time and care at first. However, flat nipples almost always improve on the way through pregnancy, and breastfeeding helps enormously. After a while, the nipples may even cease to be flat, becoming quite different from how they were before. Your ante-natal clinic may recommend *breast shells* during pregnancy to help draw out your nipples. These can help (see *inverted nipples, latching on*).

FLUID RETENTION This is quite common during pregnancy and it's usually not serious enough to warrant any special treatment (apart from extra rest). You may notice it particularly round the ankles and perhaps round the fingers and even the face. In occasional cases, it can be associated with *pre-eclampsia* or, very rarely indeed, heart or kidney disease (where there are always other symptoms) (see *oedema*).

FOLIC ACID One of the B vitamins, folic acid is particularly necessary in pregnancy as it helps in the formation of red blood cells. Folic acid is present in green leafy vegetables, and you should aim to have some every day.

FONTANELLE The 'soft spot' at the top of a baby's skull. In fact there are several soft spots, but this one, known as the anterior fontanelle, is the most obvious. The skull bones are formed during pregnancy from membrane, and the process of ossification (turning into bone) doesn't complete until after birth. There remain several gaps in the skull, which allow the baby's head to be moulded during delivery. Birth would be more difficult if the baby's skull was rigid all over. During infancy, the gaps gradually close.

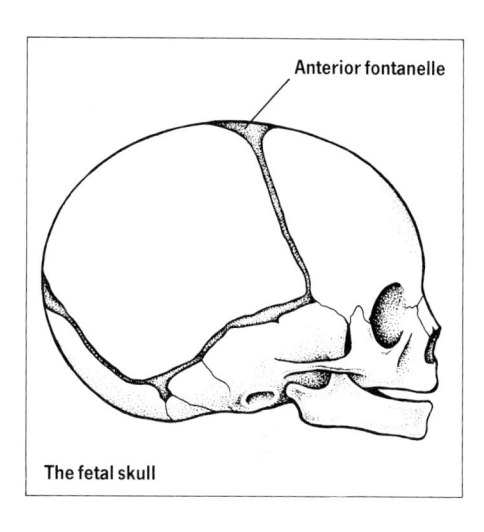

The fetal skull

FORCEPS These are instruments used to help deliver a baby towards the end of the second stage of labour. There are three main types in current use: Keilland's forceps, used when the baby's head needs to be turned; Simpson or Barnes Neville forceps, which are long, and Wrigley's forceps, which are lightweight and short. All types of forceps are shaped like a pair of curved spoons hinged together, with each blade shaped to fit the head. Doctors choose which type to use partly according to how far down the birth canal the baby is, and partly according to personal preference and what they are most practised with, and partly according to whether the head needs turning. The doctor needs to apply great skill to judge the force needed when using the forceps, and in ascertaining the correct angle to pull, to avoid damaging mother or baby. Deciding when and if to use forceps is a matter of careful judgement too. They may be used in situations when the baby's head seems unable to descend any further because of its position (as in *deep transverse arrest*) or because of the mother's

FOREWATERS

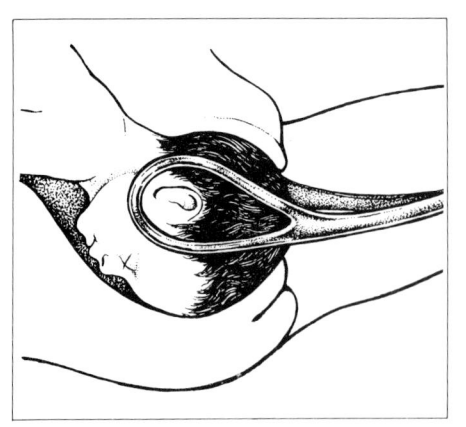

The forceps create a 'cradle' around the baby's head, allowing the doctor to help the birth of the baby's head. Forceps have a limited closing space and do not continuously squeeze the baby's head as it is gently pulled through the opening.

pelvic bones. Sometimes, the contractions become weak, or perhaps the baby shows signs of fetal distress and needs help to be born quickly. A breech baby's head may be delivered by forceps. For a forceps delivery, you are anaesthetised – either with a local or less commonly a general – and given an episiotomy. Each forceps blade is introduced separately and then hinged to the other at the handles. The doctor then gradually pulls and gently lifts. Babies delivered by forceps may have temporary bruising. Between 10 and 15 per cent of UK babies are delivered by forceps. An alternative instrument is the *ventouse*.

FOREWATERS This is the *amniotic fluid* in the womb lying in front of the baby's head (or in front of the legs or bottom if the baby is breech).

FRIENDS I don't think you can over-estimate the value of friends when you're pregnant or a new mother. And you can't over-estimate the effects of loneliness when you have a new baby as your sole daytime companion. Of course, some of us are more self-sufficient than others, and don't need other people quite so much. But everyone needs to feel valued, liked for themselves and supported – and there's only so much a partner or close relative can do. If you're used to being at work every day, you might not know anyone living near you. Even if you intend going back to work after a few months, aim to make room in your life for new friends, as your life will change when you're a parent. Ante-natal classes are an obvious way to meet others while you're still pregnant: pass a paper round the last class and ask people to put their name and address and phone number on it. The teacher may also be willing to organise a class reunion when all your babies are born. Take your courage in both hands and ring the women you warm to on the list and suggest they visit for a cup of tea one day. Of course you won't make bosom pals with everyone, but meeting as many people as you can gives you a pool from which friendships naturally develop. Lots of health clinics have mother and baby groups that meet socially; if yours doesn't, speak to a sympathetic health visitor, and see if she'll help you set one up. Most toddler groups welcome mothers with young babies as well, and the National Childbirth Trust's local branches run neighbourhood-based post-natal groups.

Making new friends, I'm convinced, helps avoid post-natal depression and your friends' children can be wonderful company for your own through infancy, toddlerhood and beyond. If you're shy, it can be a painful effort to get out and meet others – but it's worth it. Conversely if you're the chatty, garrulous sort, who finds it all very easy, reach out to the shy lonely mother who finds it cripplingly difficult. And never be afraid to ask for, or offer, help.

FSH Follicle stimulating hormone. This is a vital hormone in *conception*, released by the pituitary gland to stimulate one (or more) of the follicles in the ovary to mature, and then reach the stage where the ovum is released.

FUNDUS The top of the uterus. The height of the fundus is noted by the midwife or doctor and used as an indication or confirmation of how far on you are in your pregnancy.

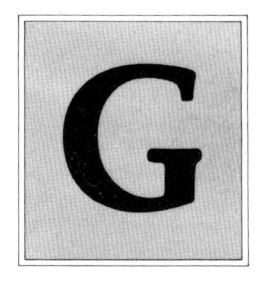

GAMMAGLOBULIN A protein in the blood which contains *antibodies*. Anti-D *gammaglobulin* is used in the prevention of *rhesus disease*.

GAS AND AIR A misnomer for a mixture of nitrous oxide and oxygen (see *Entonox*).

GENE Every cell in the body contains *chromosomes* and on the chromosomes are genes, which govern the hereditary characteristics of each individual – their blood group, height, build, hair and eye colour, for example, as well as personality traits. The only people with identical genes are identical twins.

GENERAL ANAESTHETIC The three situations which call for a general anaesthetic – when you lose consciousness – during labour and birth are a *caesarean section*, a difficult *forceps* delivery and manual removal of the placenta where the placenta fails to come away of its own accord (see *retained placenta*).

GENETIC COUNSELLING Your family doctor can refer you for genetic counselling if you are at all anxious about the possibility of becoming pregnant and passing on an inherited disease or disorder, or some sort of congenital handicap. A specialist qualified in medical genetics would then take a detailed family history from both you and your partner, possibly arranging for tests as well. In many cases, he can let you know the chances of having an affected child, but only you can make the decision to go ahead or not.

GERMAN MEASLES See *rubella*.

GLUCOSE/DEXTROSE DRIP Occasionally, a woman may have *ketones* in her urine during labour, indicating a potential lack of energy stores in her body. Hospitals usually deal with the ketones-in-the-urine situation by setting up a glucose (dextrose) drip, which feeds a sugar solution directly into your bloodstream. It's very effective, but for some women, the drip itself can be a great nuisance, because it means they are less mobile (see *eating in labour*).

GP General practitioner, also known as a family doctor and your first port of call at the start of pregnancy. He or she will see you throughout your pregnancy if you have shared ante-natal care or a home birth. All GPs are qualified to give pregnancy care and to deliver babies, but some have an extra obstetric qualification, too.

GP UNIT A General Practitioner Unit may be a small hospital delivering babies under the supervision of mothers' own GPs, or, more commonly, a unit within a larger hospital with its own 'consultant units'. GP units are normally for women expecting straightforward deliveries, and intervention is usually kept to a deliberate minimum. You will be cared for during pregnancy mainly by

GUTHRIE TEST

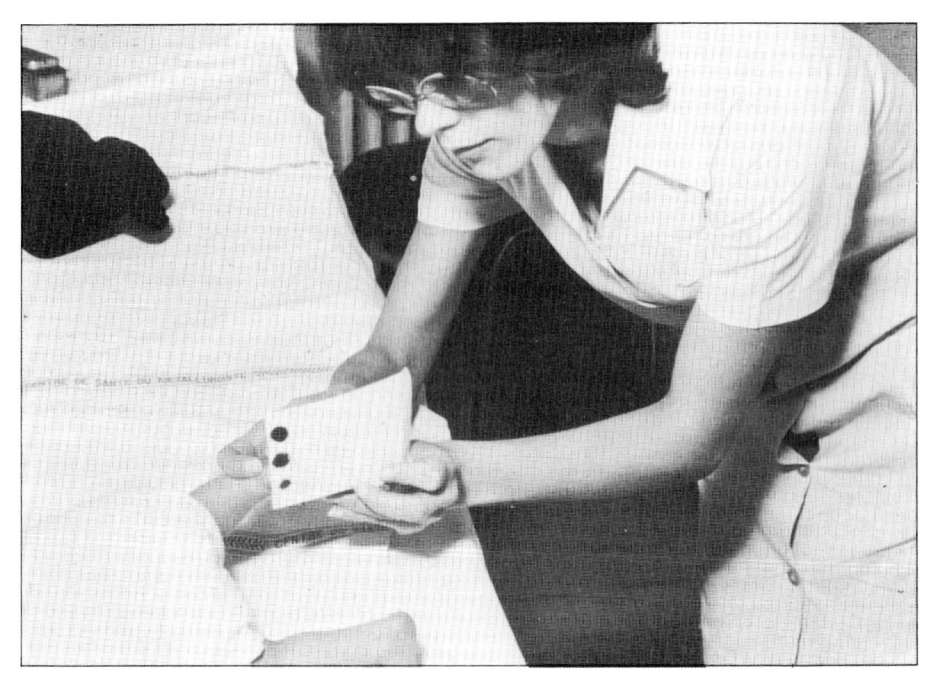

A small sample of blood is taken from the baby's heel.

the community midwife, and she may be the one who delivers you in hospital, within the GP unit. GPs vary in the amount of involvement they take on in this situation, though your GP will be informed when you are in labour, and will probably see you shortly after the birth. You are normally discharged quite soon from a GP unit, sometimes as early as 6 or 12 hours. If you want the reassurance of a hospital delivery, by feeling that specialist and emergency care is almost literally 'next door', but you want to avoid the feeling of being part of a large 'baby factory', then delivery in a GP unit may be a good choice for you (see *domino scheme*).

GUTHRIE TEST　A simple test done on a small amount of blood taken from a newborn baby's heel (usually at some time in the first week after birth). It's done to check for a rare biochemical disorder called phenylketonuria (PKU) which can lead to severe brain damage unless a special diet is followed strictly.

GYNAECOLOGIST　A doctor qualified to deal with problems concerning the female reproductive system. Gynaecologists are normally also obstetricians.

H

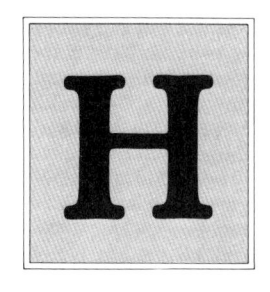

HABITUAL ABORTION See *recurrent abortion*.

HAEMOGLOBIN A compound in the red cells of the blood. Your haemoglobin level will be tested (by taking a blood sample) during pregnancy – perhaps twice, and maybe more if there's a problem. *Anaemia* shows up as a low level of haemoglobin (see *iron*).

HAEMORRHAGE A bleed. In pregnancy and labour a haemorrhage is almost always from the site of the placenta, which is normally firmly attached to the wall of the uterus. A haemorrhage, left untreated, is hazardous as the mother can lose a great deal of blood, and if the placenta ceases to nourish and support the baby, the baby's health and life are in danger too. After the baby has been born, there may occasionally be heavy bleeding from the placental site, if the blood vessels aren't closed off as a result of third stage contractions, or if there is still some placenta in the uterus. This sort of haemorrhage is known as *post-partum haemorrhage* (see *ante-partum haemorrhage*).

HAIR IN PREGNANCY During pregnancy, the normal process whereby we lose (and replace) hair every day is halted, and some women report their hair is particularly thick at this time. After childbirth, some women find the situation is reversed and they start losing hair in quite large quantities. See your doctor if this actually leaves you with thin or balding patches.

HANDICAP The vast majority of babies born are healthy and perfectly normal. In a small number there may be a handicap present at birth, sometimes a relatively minor and correctable one (a cleft lip, for instance); sometimes severe enough to be invariably fatal (for instance, *anencephaly*). The causes of many handicaps are not known, but some are inherited, and *genetic counselling* before you become pregnant may answer and deal with anxieties you may have about passing on some condition to your children. Chromosomal abnormalities like Down's syndrome show up with *amniocentesis*, and the mother is offered an abortion. Although the birth of a handicapped child can be a grave tragedy for the family, effective treatment and care can help to lessen the effects and the enormous strains. Self-help groups of affected families can give support, and many encourage research as well as persuading the rest of society to accept handicapped children and their families as part of the community.

HCG Human chorionic gonadotrophin – a hormone secreted by the fertilised egg itself. Its presence is detectable in your urine in early pregnancy, and it is HCG that's looked for in modern-day pregnancy tests. The newest tests can detect it only a few days after conception, though tests generally available in chemists are not effective until at least a day or two after your period is missed.

HEAD OF BABY A baby's head is very pliable at birth, because the bones of the skull are not yet fused together. The bones can actually slide over each other during labour and delivery, which results in some degree of 'moulding' of the head – always temporary (see *fontanelle*).

HEADACHES

HEADACHES If you suffer from frequent headaches in pregnancy, inform your doctor or ante-natal clinic. In a few cases it can be an indication of high blood pressure, though in most cases no obvious cause is found. Conscious efforts at relaxation may help, if your headaches are caused by tension. As ever, avoid medication unless prescribed by your doctor.

HEALTH BEFORE PREGNANCY Informed opinion now states it's wise to get you and your partner into good shape *before* you conceive. This 'pre-conceptual care' is thought to increase your chances of a healthy pregnancy and a healthy baby. It involves giving up smoking, any unnecessary drugs, eating well and healthily and cutting out (or down on) alcohol. Women who have been on the Pill are advised to wait at least three months after stopping before trying to conceive, to give the body a chance to return to its normal cycles. Some GPs are happy to give you advice plus a medical examination to help you assess any changes in your lifestyle that might be needed.

HEALTH DURING PREGNANCY The medical side of your pregnancy will be looked after with routine ante-natal care, but general health is much more to do with the way you look after yourself. A good varied *diet*, little or no *smoking*, little or no *alcohol*, sensible *exercise* and *rest*, no non-essential *drugs* – all these factors contribute to your general state of health. The problem can be that lack of money, lack of knowledge and lack of time conspire to make the aim of good health during pregnancy more difficult. It's important then to seek advice and help where you need it. With the right knowledge, a good diet needn't be expensive (see your hospital dietician), and friends and neighbours can take toddlers off your hands while you rest. Make sure, too, you are applying for and getting the right financial benefits during pregnancy.

HEALTH VISITOR A fully qualified nurse who has also done midwifery training, plus training in community health. Usually she'll take over the care of you and your baby from the midwife when your baby is about 10 days old though your midwife may continue to see you for longer than this. The health visitor will visit you at home initially, and maybe a few other times during your baby's first year or two. You'll be invited to telephone her if you need advice, or to ask for a home visit, and she'll encourage you to come to the *baby clinic* sessions so your baby can be weighed and to give you the chance to talk over any queries or problems. The health visitor is trained to spot any problems that need dealing with by the doctor, and she's often a useful first port-of-call if you think there may be something not-quite-right with your baby's behaviour or development. In fact, a good health visitor can be a wonderful friend and supporter, particularly to a new mother, and it's worth getting to know her well. She will also help with sleeping problems, toddler problems and anything to do with your children.

HEARTBURN A form of sickness or nausea many women get during pregnancy.

HEART OF FETUS The baby's heart starts to beat within the first month of pregnancy, and ultrasonic detectors can spot a heart beat from very early on, though at the ante-natal clinic they won't listen for the heart beat until after the 20th week or so. The midwife uses an ear trumpet or a stethoscope, and she might not be able to pick up the heart beat until about the 23rd or 24th week. In pregnancy the fetus has a heart rate of between 120 and 160 beats a minute. During labour, the fetal heart beat is monitored to check on the baby's health; a slow or inexplicably irregular rate could be a sign of fetal distress. In most hospitals today, *fetal monitors* are available which give a continuous record of the heart rate.

HEIGHT OF MOTHER Extraordinary statements sometimes pass into modern-day folklore. One of these is that if you're under 5 feet 2 inches in height you'll have to have a caesarean section. It's true that if you are small, and bearing what appears to be a large baby your pelvis may not be wide enough to allow for a safe, vaginal birth. But you may have the archetypal 'childbearing hips', or your baby may be quite the right size for you (very likely in fact), so *disproportion* doesn't arise. Small mothers show up on the statistics as being more likely to have problems generally with labour and birth, but this could be because there are more small women in social classes 4 and 5, where figures show a higher number of problems anyway.

HERPES The herpes virus causes both cold sores and infection of the genital area. The worst thing about it is that it comes back again and again, and if you are already a sufferer it may of course return during pregnancy. The danger to a baby lies in coming into contact with herpes sores around the genital area during birth. There is then a risk of brain damage, and possibly death. The solution could be to deliver the baby by caesarean section to avoid contact with any sores.

HIGH RISK This is a description from the on-the-whole worthy attempts of researchers to establish which women are more likely to have problems during pregnancy and birth, either with their own health or that of their babies. The idea is that high-risk women can be watched more carefully ante-natally, and specialist resources can be directed specifically at them, rather than spread more thinly round everyone. If you are designated high-risk you'll probably be advised to give birth in the consultant unit of a hospital (as opposed to a *GP unit* or at *home*), and the consultant may see you at each ante-natal appointment, if you are thought to be 'very' high-risk. Risk factors include previous obstetric problems (repeated miscarriage, a still birth, for example); having your first baby over the age of 30 (sometimes 35); a history of infertility; diabetes; if you are a 'grande multipara' (with four or more previous births). Most doctors won't look at isolated risk factors, however, and will take the whole picture into account. A 32 year old having a first baby, who is in otherwise very good health, for instance, is not really high-risk anywhere other than on paper. You can become high-risk during pregnancy, if, for example, it's discovered you're having twins (or more), if your baby seems *light-for-dates* or not in an ideal position.

HIGH TECH Applied to childbirth, this describes an approach favouring intervention and aids like the fetal monitor, ultrasound and epidurals. In fact, most doctors – and mothers – would agree that of course technology has a place. The argument is about how enthusiastic we should be about its wider application (see *Savage, Wendy*).

HOME BIRTH Before the second world war, most babies were born at home. Through the 1960s, a policy of encouraging hospital births took off, and maternity bed provision was made with this in mind. The result is today that if you want to have your baby in hospital, you have no problem. In fact, your problems can begin if you don't. One estimate is that only about 2 per cent of babies are born at home these days though the figure may be higher. In some areas, there are even fewer home deliveries, as the run down of the community midwifery services has paralleled the increase in maternity bed provision (and home deliveries are normally carried out by community midwives). As fewer babies are born at home, the midwives themselves get fewer chances to deliver babies, and some may actually feel a bit 'rusty', and encourage mothers to opt for hospital on this basis. The gap between the sort of emergency facilities available in a home setting, and the high-tech equipment (for resuscitating babies with breathing problems, for instance) in hospitals means that in an emergency the hospital is better able to act quickly and effectively. However, some authorities are acknowledging that policies of intervention and medical control of labour (induction, acceleration, zealous use of drugs) in hospital actually bring their own hazards to normal birth. Home could in fact be the safer place for some women. Recent research shows a very low peri-natal mortality rate for home birth, compared with hospital. Up-to-date research is needed now which compares the outcomes of a sufficiently high number of planned home deliveries, with a matched sample of planned hospital deliveries, choosing maternity units who deliberately avoid unnecessary intervention, and who expressly allow choice of position in labour and delivery and so on. Results from this sort of study would give a clearer overall picture, as the low peri-natal mortality rate at home must at least partly reflect the fact that home-booked mothers tend to be from the higher social groups – which have a better pregnancy outcome anyway.

Nevertheless, the home versus hospital debate hasn't revolved round statistics. It's been about the depersonalisation of childbirth. At home, a mother feels in control. Any medical attendants are there as visitors. She isn't separated from her familiar environment and she feels secure. For a woman with no medical or obstetric reason to expect anything other than a normal birth, these advantages may outweigh everything else and of course they can't really be quantified or evaluated in statistical terms (neither can happiness or joy, or calmness – all feelings which some mothers may find more 'achievable' at home).

If you decide a home birth is for you, remember you have a legal right to it. Your first step is to contact your GP. He will help evaluate the medical side of the equation for you (although, of course, he may have his own strong feelings for or against home birth, and you will soon be aware what these are). If he is prepared to go along with your wishes, fine. If not, you can transfer to another GP for the duration of your pregnancy. If you can't find a GP to support you, your health authority is still under a statutory obligation to provide midwifery care for you at home. You should in that case write to your local district nursing officer, asking for this midwifery care, and pointing out that your GP does not wish you to have a home birth.

There are categories of women who really are better off in hospital, and that doesn't just include the 'high-risk' ones. If your housing situation is overcrowded, or without easy access to running hot water, for instance, then you may well be more comfortable in hospital. If you have no one to look after you immediately after the birth, too, a hospital stay is the only way you'll get the rest you need (see *hospital birth*, Useful Addresses).

HOME HELP A service run by the local authority to help the elderly, disabled or sick, plus mothers of young children, with household tasks. If you've been ill during pregnancy, or if you have children born close together, it's worth asking about having a home help. You may be required to contribute to the cost, according to your income.

HORMONES The definition often given in school biology lessons is a useful one here: hormones are 'chemical messengers'. They are produced in one part of the body and then sent through the bloodstream to another part, and this other part reacts in a certain way to the presence of this hormone. During pregnancy, specific hormones are made that are produced at no other time, or if they are, in different quantities. The major production of pregnancy hormones is undertaken by the placenta. After the baby is born, hormones are produced by the action of breastfeeding and they cause the production of and the release of milk.

HOSPITAL BIRTH By far the majority of babies (98 per cent) are born in hospital in the UK, yet hospital birth has had something of a bad press in recent years. However, if we define good maternity care as being based on

HOSPITAL BIRTH

a willingness to listen to and to act on an individual's wishes, rather than according to hospital or consultant policy, then evidence shows that some progress is being made, albeit in a patchy sort of way. There still seems to be a wide gap between firstly, the hospital that seems to do its very best to treat its mothers as people rather than patients, happy to learn about new ideas on pregnancy and childbirth and relaxed in its dealings with women before, during and after birth, and secondly the sort of regulation NHS-issue Bloggsville General, with its long ante-natal clinic queues, impersonal treatment, rigid routines and automatic interventions. The lack of choice in many parts of the country means that many women are destined to give birth at Bloggsville General. Women themselves can help the situation, by creating a demand for the services they want, by not being nervous about discussing their needs and wishes at the ante-natal clinic. For instance, you may know you want an epidural, or an early discharge, or you may want to avoid an episiotomy, so *tell* the medical staff at the clinic. If you aren't very good at putting over your feelings, take someone with you to back you up.

The main – and not inconsiderable – advantage of a hospital birth is that emergency facilities and specialist knowledge are on the spot should anything go wrong with the birth, or in the period immediately after. For many women, this gives peace of mind and confidence.

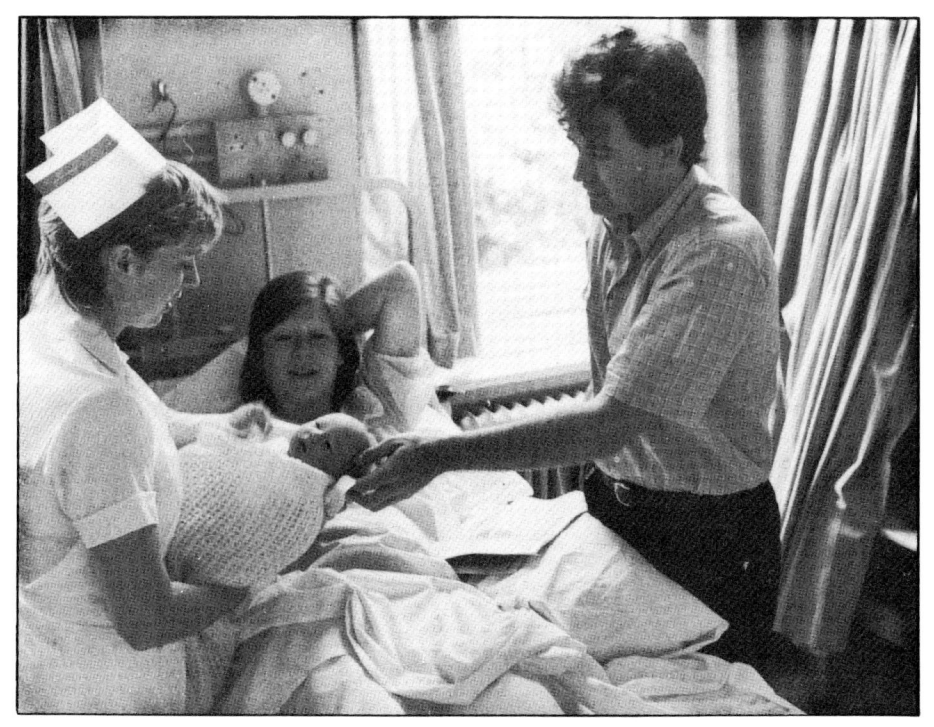

One advantage of having your baby in hospital is that medical and nursing help is at hand to give advice and support when needed.

HOSPITAL DISCHARGE

HOSPITAL DISCHARGE   Different hospitals have different recommendations as to when it's advisable to go home after having your baby. As a rule, mothers having first babies stay in for five days or more; second and subsequent timers are discharged after 48 hours. If there has been any departure from the norm (for example, caesarean, forceps, post-partum haemorrhage) you may be advised to stay a bit longer, mainly so you and/or the baby can continue to be observed. If your baby needs special care, you would be unlikely to be able to stay with him in hospital for many days at a time (although some *special care* units have beds available for mothers to use, stays of many weeks would be discouraged as beds are likely to be limited).

If you want to be discharged earlier than the hospital's usual policy, this can usually be arranged, though it makes things easier for everyone if you ask in advance (and of course no one could keep you in hospital against your will – it's not a prison!). In areas with a shortage of community midwives (who are the ones who look after you when you get home) early discharge may not be looked on very favourably.

Think about what you want from a hospital stay before you have your baby. You may enjoy the break from home, using the time to learn about caring for your baby and getting to know her. And if you're the anxious sort, you get on-the-spot advice and reassurance in hospital. The spirit of togetherness and mutual support you get between mothers on the post-natal wards can be a good and valuable experience, too. On the other hand, you may long to get back to your own bed, and if you have other children you may not want to be parted from them. Make sure you'll have the chance to do nothing except look after the baby if you want to be home earlier though; this will mean getting someone to do all the household tasks and shopping.

HOSPITAL GOWN   It may be hospital policy to issue you with a hospital gown to wear for your labour and delivery. It's only a small point, but if you find out that this is the case, then ask if you can bring in two clean nighties of your own. They will at least fit you, you will feel more comfortable in something of your own, and they won't be open down the back like most hospital gowns are. This is important, as if you intend to move around in labour you may feel self-conscious in an unattractive and yet almost totally revealing garment. If you use your own nighties be prepared for them to get into a bit of a mess, or even spoilt, so don't choose your best ones.

HOSPITAL NURSERY   Each post-natal ward usually has its own warm, well-lit nursery. In the past babies were kept there most of the time, and taken to their mothers for feeding. Now this era is passing, and most babies stay with their mothers in cribs next to their beds. You might be asked to put your baby in the nursery at night, but you may prefer not to do this. If he's beside you, you will be able to tend to him immediately if he wakes (see *rooming-in*).

HOSPITAL STAFF   At the ante-natal clinic, you're likely to see midwives (both student and 'staff' – qualified) and possibly general nurses as well. You'll probably also see doctors: they can be SHOs (senior house officers), usually youngish qualified doctors getting some 'obs and gynae' practice before deciding what branch of medicine to specialise in. Above these in the medical hierarchy are registrars and senior registrars, who have already decided to make specialist careers in obstetrics and gynaecology, and who may have several years' experience. Right at the top is the consultant. You'll be assigned to a consultant (or maybe a senior registrar) when you book in at the hospital ante-natal clinic, though if all goes well you might not see him. The doctors are known as Mr (or Miss or Mrs) somebody-or-other if they are also qualified surgeons. If they are physicians, they are Dr somebody-or-other. If a midwife is 'sister', she is especially senior and experienced, and may, for example, be in charge of the nursing side of an ante-natal

HYDATIDIFORM MOLE

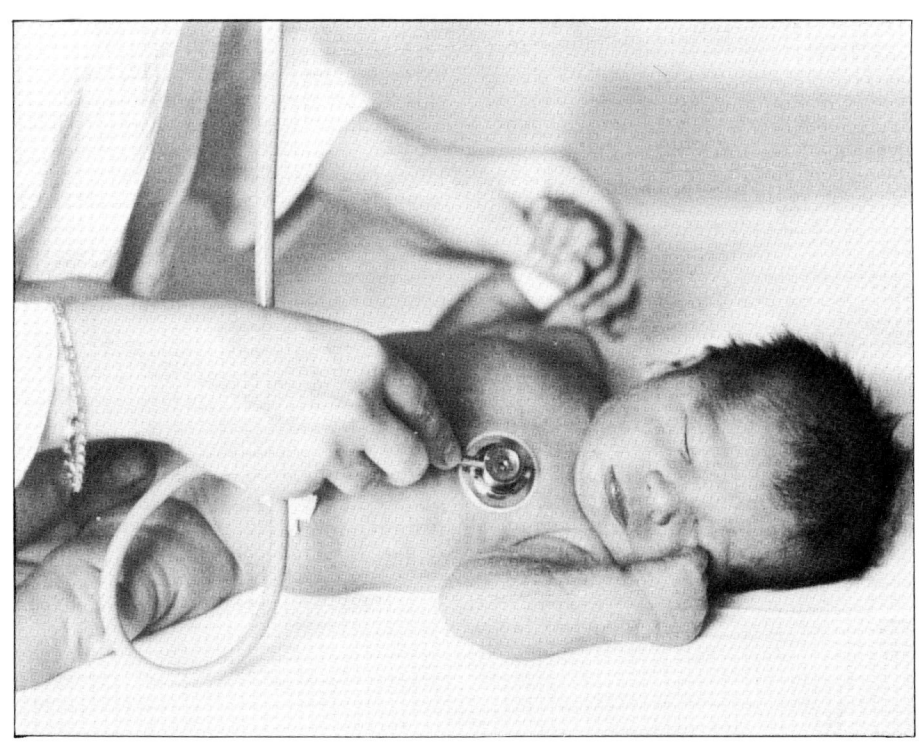

A paediatrician will check your baby soon after the birth.

clinic or a labour or post-natal ward. After the birth you may meet a paediatrician – a specialist in child health – and/or Senior House Officers (SHOs) doing a paediatric stint.

I think it would be nice if everybody you met during your pregnancy and birth could do you the small courtesy of introducing themselves. And it would be a welcome change if you could see the same small team of carers throughout. This would mean re-organisation, as at present obstetric care is neatly parcelled into three – ante-natal care, labour and birth, post-natal care. It's only women having babies at home who can rely on anything approaching continuity.

HYDATIDIFORM MOLE A hydatidiform mole pregnancy arises when the fertilised egg fails to develop, and the embryo is absorbed into the body at around the sixth week. However the chorionic villii which are attached to the wall of the uterus start to grow little grape-like sacs. These sacs proliferate and eventually fill the uterus. There's no longer any pregnancy, but pregnancy hormones are still made and so you still have no periods, you still have tender breasts and you may still feel sick. The outcome of hydatidiform mole is always the loss of the contents of the uterus, beginning with vaginal bleeding. Hospital admission is always needed, to make sure the uterus is cleared, and to ensure prompt treatment for haemorrhage (which can happen with this sort of *miscarriage*).

HYDROCEPHALY/HYDROCEPHALUS
(*hy-dro-kéff-aly/hy-dro-kéff-alluss*) A serious condition resulting from an excess of cerebrospinal fluid, which is the fluid the body produces to bathe the brain and spinal cord. Hydrocephaly is seen on its own or commonly with *spina bifida*. The most obvious symptom is a gross enlargement of the head in a new baby, or in an infant. The condition is dealt with by surgically draining the skull, and this treatment can be quite successful (though if left untreated, brain damage, and possibly death, may result).

HYGIENE
Hospitals are the germiest places to be – far more bug-ridden than your average home – which is why everyone makes a special effort to observe strict rules of cleanliness during labour and birth and afterwards. However, although little babies don't have the same resistance to infection as a healthy adult, and you do need to maintain certain minimum standards at home, hospital rules needn't apply. So, even if you've done so in hospital, you don't need sterile cotton wool to wash your baby's face. Nevertheless always wash your hands after changing his nappy; clean his face before his bottom – and let common sense rather than obsession, rule! If you're bottle feeding, though, you'll need to be strict about sterilising.

HYPERTENSION
The medical term for high *blood pressure*.

HYPERVENTILATION
This is also termed 'overbreathing'. It can sometimes happen in the late first stage of labour as a result of taking in too much oxygen, by breathing in too quickly and not letting out sufficient air. You therefore upset the oxygen/carbon dioxide balance of your body. It's not harmful, but you can feel uncomfortably dizzy and tingling. The remedy is simple: breathe more gently and concentrate carefully on the out breath. You can also cup your hands over your nose and face for a few breaths.

HYPNOSIS
An alternative method of pain-relief in labour that you prepare for during pregnancy under the guidance of a specially trained person. You are taught to achieve a semi-trance like state which blocks the pain of contractions. You don't lose consciousness at all and you're perfectly aware of everything going on around you. It's more a sort of ability to distance yourself from your contractions. If you think hypnosis would be right for you, you'll need to see a hypnotherapist with a special interest in childbirth preparation.

HYPOGLYCAEMIA
Low blood sugar level, sometimes seen in a pre-term or light-for-dates newborn. It usually shows up as 'jittery' movements. Treatment is simple: sugar is given to the baby, orally or perhaps via a drip, and normal milk feeding continues.

HYPOSPADIAS
A fairly rare abnormality present at birth in boys. The urethra (the opening leading from the bladder) doesn't end at the tip of the penis, but on the underside. In cases where the opening is very near the tip surgery might not be necessary, but in most cases an operation (or operations) are needed. The outlook is usually very good.

I

INCOMPETENT CERVIX A medical phrase which sounds very derogatory to the lay person, but which isn't meant to be taken personally. It refers to the cervix which won't stay closed for the duration of pregnancy. The result is usually a late miscarriage, with the woman's cervix dilating, her waters perhaps breaking and the inevitable loss of her baby. Once cervical incompetence has been diagnosed after one or more late miscarriages the treatment is usually a purse string stitch (called a *Shirodkar stitch*) inserted in early pregnancy to keep the cervix closed. It's removed in later pregnancy, or earlier if labour begins sooner.

INCOMPLETE ABORTION This happens when you've had a miscarriage, but not all the 'products of conception' have come away. It's sometimes possible for there to be some retention in the uterus of the placenta, or part of the placenta. The main danger is haemorrhage, and this will be treated before the rest of the pregnancy is taken away surgically.

INCUBATOR A special crib for sick or low birthweight babies. It's kept at a very warm, even temperature as tiny babies can't regulate their own body temperatures. An increased concentration of oxygen can be introduced into the incubator if needed. Linked to the incubator may be machines to monitor breathing and heart rate (see *special care*).

INDUCTION This describes any process which starts labour off artificially, and there are various methods. The simplest way is for the membranes holding the amniotic fluid to be pierced (*artificial rupture of the membranes – ARM*). This often starts the uterus contracting (most likely in a woman who would be likely to deliver spontaneously within a few days). At the same time as ARM, or more usually later if nothing has happened, an artificial hormone drip may be set up which puts a dose of synthetic *oxytocin* directly into the bloodstream. This causes the uterus to start contracting. The level of pressure inside the uterus is assessed throughout the labour, sometimes by the midwife, sometimes by a specially developed machine linked via a tube to the inside of the uterus, and the dosage of oxytocin is regulated accordingly.

Induction can also be done with *prostaglandin* pessaries, which are inserted high up in the vagina (though a drip and ARM may follow the use of pessaries if labour doesn't appear to be getting underway), where it melts and releases the substance which starts the uterus contracting.

Another (fairly simple) method of induction is a 'membrane sweep' (or a 'stretch and sweep'): the membranes are stretched and separated from the lower part of the uterus, and this seems to stimulate the cervix, and thence the uterus, into contracting.

Methods and combinations of methods of induction have been a rich field of research, as doctors have evaluated them from the point of view of length of labour, efficiency of contractions and effect on the baby, as well as trying to find out whether one method or another is more, or less, likely to lead to further intervention.

There are certain medical indications for induction. These can affect the mother, or the baby, or both. If you have *pre-eclampsia* or *high blood pressure*, or *diabetes*, for example, it may be considered that your baby's better out than

INFERTILITY

in. Similarly, if it's thought your baby's no longer being well-nourished because the placenta has stopped working (*placental insufficiency*) or if he's showing signs of distress (slow heart rate, lack of movement) labour could be induced. The real areas of controversy though aren't within these categories. One of them is about *post-maturity*. Many obstetricians induce after 41 weeks of pregnancy to avoid post-maturity, but whether this factor justifies the intervention of induction, and how far you can avoid inducing babies who aren't 42 weeks but who are really 38 weeks (because a miscalculation of dates can sometimes arise) is not clear. Some recent work has been done with so-called 'oxytocin-challenge tests', where the mother of a supposedly post-mature fetus is given small doses of oxytocin, then taken off the hormone. The fetus is assessed (through monitoring, looking at the amniotic fluid, checking movement) to gauge how it has responded to the challenge of contractions. If it doesn't respond well, labour is induced. If there appears to be no problem, pregnancy is allowed to continue. Again, it's not clear how far this work will go or how tolerant mothers would be of this procedure.

Induction as a whole has undergone a fairly radical reassessment in the last few years. Ten or fifteen years ago, induction was more common than it is now, and newspapers 'exposed' the disturbing trend of inductions undertaken for reasons more connected with staffing levels and convenience than medical necessity. At the time, it wasn't uncommon for women to be induced at an hour of the day when staff would be around, at a time of the week (i.e. not Saturday or Sunday) convenient to the doctor. There were claims that mothers were induced to fit in with the consultant's private work or even his golf competitions. This tendency is no longer obvious, and if it still exists anywhere it's not readily admitted to. Currently inductions run at about 10 to 15 per cent of all deliveries, and obstetricians are keener than they were to make sure the advantages of induction are seen to outweigh the disadvantages in any individual case.

And disadvantages there are. Apart from the hazard of inadvertently delivering a baby not yet ready to be born (mentioned above), there is some evidence that induced babies are more likely to suffer breathing difficulties at birth; there seems to be a connection between neo-natal *jaundice* and induction; induced labours are more likely to be more painful – contractions are longer and stronger than in spontaneous labour, without the gradual build-up most women get, so mothers are more likely to need pain relief to cope (with attendant hazards to the baby); induction via a drip means that a mother is restricted in her movements, and this in its turn prevents a change of position which could help her cope with any pain.

There should always be a clear benefit whenever induction is carried out, and when induction is suggested to you, you should be given the chance to understand and appreciate the benefits to you and/or your baby.

INFERTILITY It's been estimated that one in seven couples have problems conceiving a child; most of these go on to become pregnant, some with medical help, some without. Unless you have a good reason for suspecting that either you or your partner is sub-fertile (very irregular periods, a known low-sperm count) or unless you're in your mid to late thirties when time isn't really on your side, there's little point in seeing a doctor before you've been having regular intercourse for at least six months, and possibly a year, as time, in so many cases, does the trick. Don't forget, though, your most fertile time is at or around ovulation – approximately 14 days before you expect your next period. So it makes sense to have intercourse then if you are trying for a baby.

INSOMNIA Usually more of a problem in late pregnancy, when repeated visits to the lavatory, together with your enlarged tummy, may combine to keep you awake. Make sure you're comfortable in bed: lie on your side

INTERNAL EXAMINATION

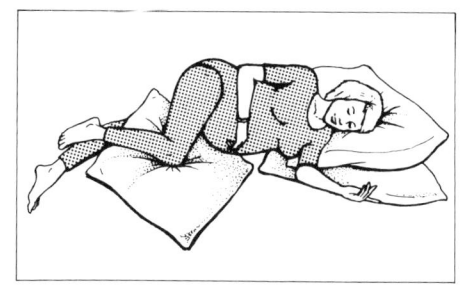

Try using cushions to support your limbs and enlarging abdomen and get more comfortable.

(with a cushion or pillow under your bump) with the upper leg flexed. Try gradually relaxing your body from the toes up and breathe deeply. A warm milk drink before you go to bed may also help.

INTENSIVE CARE Newborn babies who are born too early, or who are sick, or both, may need intensive care. Some hospitals have intensive care baby units; others have intensive care cots within the *special care* baby units. Intensive care is similar to special care but it involves more specialised and complex treatment. Neo-natal specialists have recently criticised financial stringency and low staffing levels, which mean intensive care is unavailable to all babies who need it. In some cases death or handicap is the result.

INTERCOURSE 'Is sex safe during pregnancy?' – the old question, and one which in 99 cases out of 100, has the answer 'yes'. If you are in any doubt at all, though, ask your doctor or midwife. If you've a history of miscarriage or of difficult pregnancies, then there may be a case for avoiding intercourse in the first three months at the time your period would have been due, for instance, but generally speaking having sex when you want is good for you. When your tummy gets large you may need to find positions that don't let you feel squashed, not because you might harm the baby, but because it's simply

uncomfortable. It's quite normal to find your sex drive is different in pregnancy – some women find they don't want sex so often as before; others find the opposite. Either is normal. Where there are no problems, intercourse late in pregnancy can even help to 'ripen' the cervix for delivery because of naturally occurring prostaglandins (hormone-like substances) in the semen (see *orgasm*).

INTERNAL EXAMINATION During an 'internal' or 'V.E.' (vaginal examination), your doctor or midwife can check on the size and shape of your uterus by putting one or two fingers of one hand into the vagina (to feel the cervix and lower part of the uterus) and the other hand on your tummy (to feel the uterus through the abdominal wall). He may use a speculum during the same examination. This is a metal or plastic instrument to hold the walls of the vagina apart while the doctor takes a look at the cervix, and perhaps takes a cervical smear for analysis. You may have an internal done at the beginning of pregnancy, and the other at around 36 weeks (which is primarily to check for *disproportion*).

During labour you'll be given an internal examination on admission and every so often thereafter (routine practice is about every four hours). This lets the midwife see how far the cervix has dilated. You'll probably also have

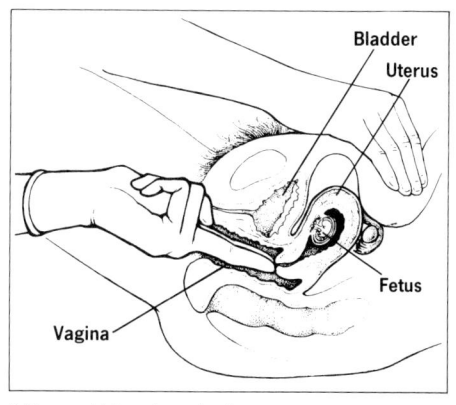

A bi-manual internal examination.

an internal at your post-natal check, six weeks or so after the birth. Internals shouldn't hurt, and if they are done gently, and you are relaxed, they won't. One way to relax yourself is to lie on the couch with your knees pointing upwards and your feet a couple of feet apart. Then allow your knees to flop apart without tensing your muscles. (If you always wear a dress rather than trousers when you expect an internal, you won't feel quite so undressed.)

INTRA-UTERINE DEATH The death of a baby still in the womb. This obviously results in *stillbirth*.

INVERTED NIPPLES Some women have nipples that don't stand out at all; they may even turn inwards like a dimple. If one or both your nipples is like this, it doesn't mean you won't be able to breastfeed, though you may need a bit of extra help. Pregnancy itself seems to cure many apparently inverted nipples, and breastfeeding improves them still further. Your midwife may recommend you to wear *breast shells* during pregnancy. A nipple shield worn while feeding can help too. Some nipples, however, are so very inverted, that coupled with a baby who doesn't suck very well, normal breastfeeding becomes too difficult. Fortunately, this is very rare.

INVOLUTION OF UTERUS This describes the return to the non-pregnant state that the uterus achieves in the days and weeks after childbirth. The muscle tissue of the uterus is broken down and dispersed harmlessly through the body, and the blood supply to the uterus is reduced. When involution isn't taking place at the rate it should, it can mean some of the placenta has been left behind, or there may be some infection present. This is why your midwife checks the size of your uterus daily after your baby is born. It's worth knowing that breastfeeding helps stimulate hormones that help the uterus reduce in size more quickly than otherwise.

IRON You need an adequate intake of iron during pregnancy to prevent iron deficiency anaemia. You could take supplements in the form of iron tablets (given out routinely in many clinics), but iron is found quite naturally in wholemeal bread, liver, kidneys, red meats, dark green vegetables and dried fruits. Routine iron supplements are thought by some experts to be not only unnecessary, but potentially even harmful, as it could be that too much iron interferes with the body's ability to absorb other minerals, notably zinc.

ITCHING IN PREGNANCY Some women are unlucky enough to experience this as a considerable nuisance all the way through pregnancy, though it almost always disappears after delivery. It's not known what causes it, but the doctor can prescribe bland creams to relieve it. Make sure you aren't wearing anything next to your skin that could be contributing to the irritation.

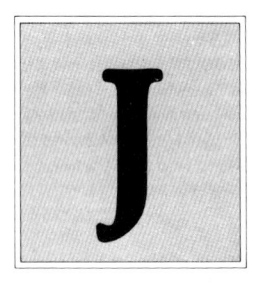

J

JAUNDICE Jaundice results in a marked yellowish skin tinge and it's rare in pregnancy, though when it happens it can be serious. Jaundice in the newborn baby is an entirely different situation. It's really very common, especially in pre term babies. Again, it shows up in the skin (seen easily in white babies) and in the whites of the eyes. In the vast majority of cases there is nothing to be anxious about at all. Newborn babies' livers are rather immature, and they may not be able to cope with breaking down excess red blood cells, and excreting the bilirubin waste product that follows the breaking down. The bilirubin remains in the body, staining the tissues yellow. A typical case of this physiological or neo-natal jaundice starts in the first few days after birth and gradually disappears without treatment over a week or so. As jaundice that becomes severe can, in occasional cases, indicate something more seriously wrong, your baby may have tests to assess his true level of jaundice, and he may be placed under special lights that speed up the breakdown of the yellow pigment.

The main problem with neo-natal jaundice is that it can make the baby sleepy and reluctant to feed. This can sometimes make the establishment of breastfeeding more difficult, but the problem almost always passes.

In rare cases, the baby may eventually be diagnosed as having 'breast milk jaundice', thought to be caused by some unknown substance in the mother's milk (though that doesn't explain why siblings escape it). The usual reaction of doctors these days is to recommend continuing breastfeeding, while the baby has outpatient's appointments for the progress or otherwise of the jaundice to be observed. This sort of jaundice is harmless though the yellow colour persists for some weeks.

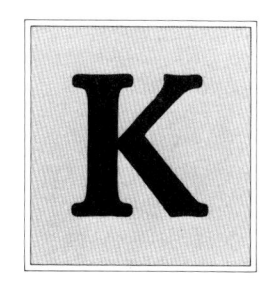

KETONES These are formed in the body as a result of ketosis, which can happen in labour, when the carbohydrate stores in the body have run out, and fat stores are being used instead. Ketones can be detected in the urine of a woman in labour, and urine is tested for this at regular intervals. If ketones build up in the body, labour can slow down, as the body chemistry is disturbed. The usual solution to ketosis is to give a sugar-solution drip, though this has the disadvantage of immobilising a woman (unless she wants to push a drip stand about with her) and keeping her in or near the bed (see *eating in labour*).

KICK CHART If your ante-natal clinic wants to check the well-being of your unborn baby for some reason, you may be given a kick chart to take home with you. On it, you usually have to make a note of your baby's movements when you feel them each morning. When you've noticed ten movements (for example) you make a note of the time by the clock, and your clinic then judges how active your baby is over a period of time. There'd be cause for concern if your baby's movements slowed down significantly or stopped altogether for some time. Doctors are still working out the most efficient method of helping mothers to record kicks without causing them undue anxiety (see *fetal movements, quickening*).

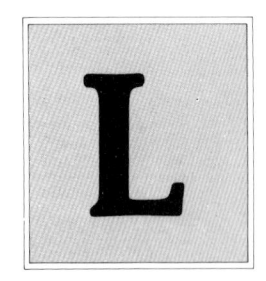

LABOUR Labour is divided into three stages by most obstetricians: the *first stage*, during which the cervix gradually opens (dilates) to let the baby through into the birth canal; the *second stage*, during which the baby is pushed down the birth canal to the outside world; and finally the *third stage*, during which the placenta is delivered.

First labours are generally longer than subsequent ones. Labour starts, on average, 40 weeks after the first day of the last period, but it can be difficult to pinpoint the exact time spontaneous labour begins. Lots of women get a day or two's warning of the start in the form of a *show* or a slight backache, or the odd twinge. The usual way of defining the start though is to mark it from the beginning of strong, regular uterine contractions, even though you may have been having labour contractions that aren't so strong, or so frequent, for some hours before this. In other cases, labour can start very quickly. It might begin with the waters breaking, followed by strong rapid contractions. If you're having a normal pregnancy, and there's no reason for you to need medical care from the start of labour, it's a good idea to stay at home for a good part of the first stage of labour unless your waters break, when you should aim to get to hospital sooner. During the day, it's easiest to keep on the move, resting when you feel the need to. At night, you can walk up and down if you can't sleep at all, make a hot drink, sit and read. If you feel happier heading for the labour ward, though, then don't worry about turning up 'too soon'. No one will mind. Labour has been likened to walking up a very steep mountain. Sometimes, the peak is obscured as you climb, but you keep on going and it soon comes into view again. The birth of your baby is at the top of the mountain, when you can rest, feeling exhilarated and suddenly refreshed. This analogy, is, I think, fairly accurate for the majority of women having a normal labour. It has to be added that labour is painful for most women, too, but the strength of that pain, the length of it, and your reaction to it, will be different from another woman's. Labour is always a great physical event, stretching you to the limits of your energy. But with the right support, confidence in ourselves, and in the people looking after us, that very event can be spiritually enriching; giving birth – even after a long and difficult labour – can be a loving, gentle act, that allows us to see a new depth and meaning in life.

The problem can be that thinking of birth in this way can make women who want the whole thing over and done with as quickly and as forgettably as possible feel resentful and guilty. After all, we may have different feelings about labour and birth, and yet most of us end up loving our babies fiercely and protectively, however we feel about their entrance into the world. But maybe it isn't quite as simple as that. *Post-natal depression* and relationship problems are often considered to be linked with a bad experience of labour. Perhaps the way forward is to help women decide how they want their babies to be born (epidural, natural, active and so on), to keep them involved at all times, so that nothing is 'done to' them, that in weeks, months or even years to come, will make them feel angry, resentful or even guilty (see *birth, bonding, pain in labour*).

LABOUR COMPANION The person you choose to be with you in labour; if you feel you need someone apart from your midwife and doctor, and many women do, this is most likely to be your partner. He can give you loving support and encouragement when you

LABOUR

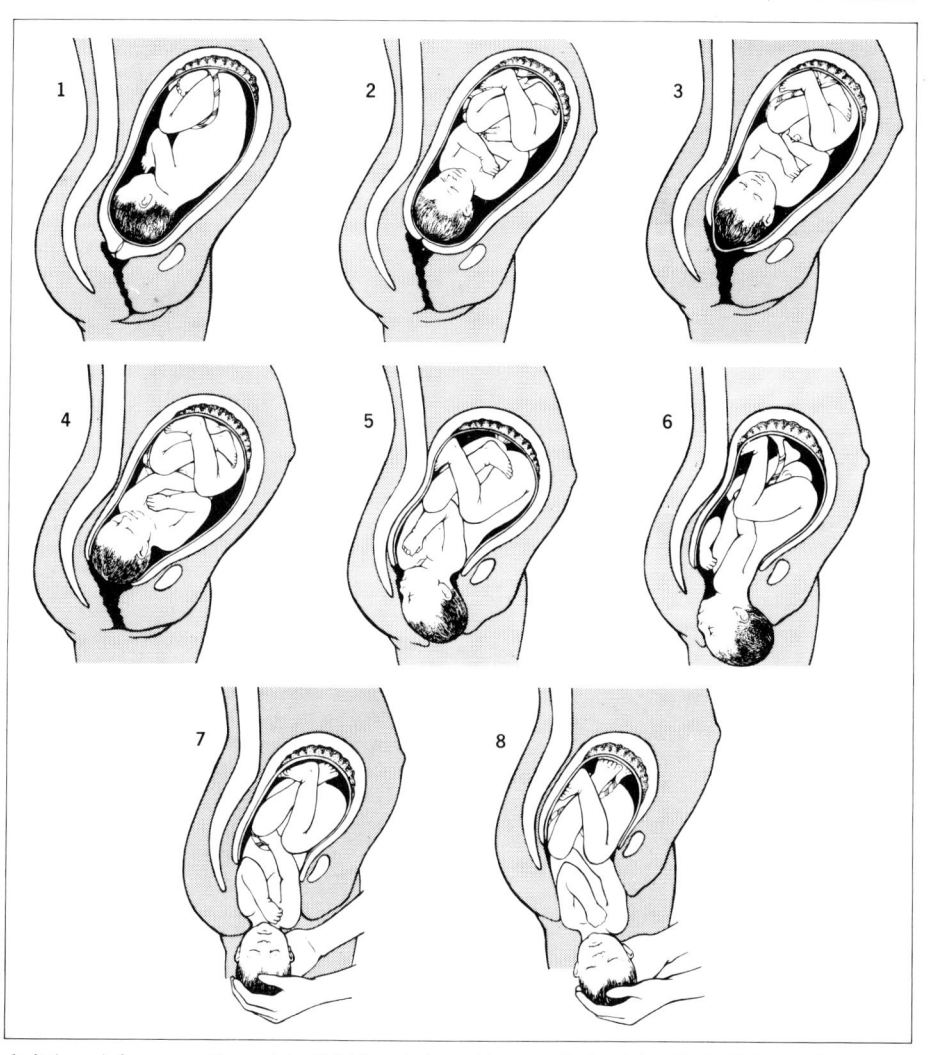

1 At the end of pregnancy, the cervix is still tightly sealed.
2 Labour starts with the cervix softening, and the mucus plug sealing the cervix comes away. The baby turns slightly, ready to descend.
3 The membranes enclosing the amniotic fluid bulge in front of the baby's head. The cervix continues to dilate to allow the head to pass (in some labours the amniotic fluid has already leaked out by this time, and in a few cases the membranes may remain intact for longer).
4 The membranes have ruptured, and the cervix is fully taken up as the baby's head begins its journey down the birth canal.
5 The baby is about to be born. The head appears (called 'crowning') and the soft bones of the baby's skull allow it to be 'moulded'.
6 The brow and head are fully born.
7 At the moment of delivery, the baby turns which allows the shoulders to be born smoothly and easily.
8 The rest of the baby is born, gently eased and guided into the world by the hands of the midwife.

LABOUR WARD

need it, and help in practical ways like bringing you water on a sponge, and by massaging you. He can also share in the joy of the birth. But it may not be possible for him to be there (he may be away or not around any more) or you may not want him there. In this case you might think about having someone else you trust and feel close to – a relative or good friend. Most hospitals are happy enough now about having fathers in the delivery room, but not all of them are used to having other people instead, so you should tell the ante-natal clinic your plans first. Mothers choosing a home birth have a greater flexibility about who is and isn't with them, but again you should still talk over the situation with your midwife (see *fathers*).

LABOUR WARD You are admitted to the labour ward when you go into hospital to have your baby. Some hospitals put women in one room for the first stage of labour, and then move them for delivery. In other hospitals women remain in one room throughout. Staying in the same place is usually less disturbing, being put on to a trolley at the end of first stage is uncomfortable and disorientating, as is having to get used to another four walls (see *delivery room*).

LACTATION The production of milk by the breasts (see *breastfeeding*).

LANUGO A fluffy sort of downy hair seen on the skin of new babies, particularly pre-term babies. It soon disappears.

LATCHING ON A *breastfeeding* term – latching on describes what a baby does when he's positioned well as the breast; it's also known as being 'fixed'. A baby who is well latched on will be able to suck well, without chomping on the end of your nipple and making it sore. In this way you will build up a good milk supply and your baby will get enough to satisfy his hunger and thirst. Avoiding sore nipples by making sure your baby's well latched on goes a long way towards making the whole breastfeeding experience a good one, in fact. Encourage your baby to fix well from the start by holding him with his face close to your breast. If you stroke his cheek he will open his mouth in readiness – a wide open mouth will cover the whole nipple and much of the surrounding areola top and bottom. It can take time for all this to come exactly right – breastfeeding is often best appreciated as a learning process, and lots of mothers need help at first.

LEBOYER, FREDERIC French obstetrician and advocate of 'gentle birth'. In a Leboyer birth, the baby is born calmly into a softly-lit, quiet room and immediately soothed in a warm bath. The ideas behind this are that 'normal' birth is traumatic and distressing to the baby. Leboyer-type principles have influenced much of today's thinking on childbirth, but the emphasis most easily detected now has already shifted – to the mother's feelings, and her participation in labour and delivery decisions.

LENGTH OF LABOUR First time labours are said on average to last between 10 and 15 hours. Second and subsequent ones are shorter. There are wide variations and a labour lasting a lot longer than 'the average' needn't always bring problems, though it may be exhausting for the mother. Most obstetricians would want to be quite sure labour was progressing well, however, with no maternal or fetal distress. Steps would otherwise be taken to speed things up or to get the baby out, by *acceleration* or *caesarean section* (or possibly *forceps* if second stage looked as if it was held up in some way) (see *labour*).

LENGTH OF PREGNANCY Pregnancy, on average, lasts 40 weeks from the first day of your last menstrual period (about 38 weeks from conception). If your periods are normally less than 28 days apart, conception will probably have taken place sooner in your cycle than the 14th day, and your expected date of delivery will be calculated to take this into account. Similarly, if you have a long cycle, your EDD will reflect a probable earlier conception. Most babies arrive within two weeks of their EDD. Twins tend to arrive sooner – the average twin pregnancy lasts 37 weeks.

LATCHING ON

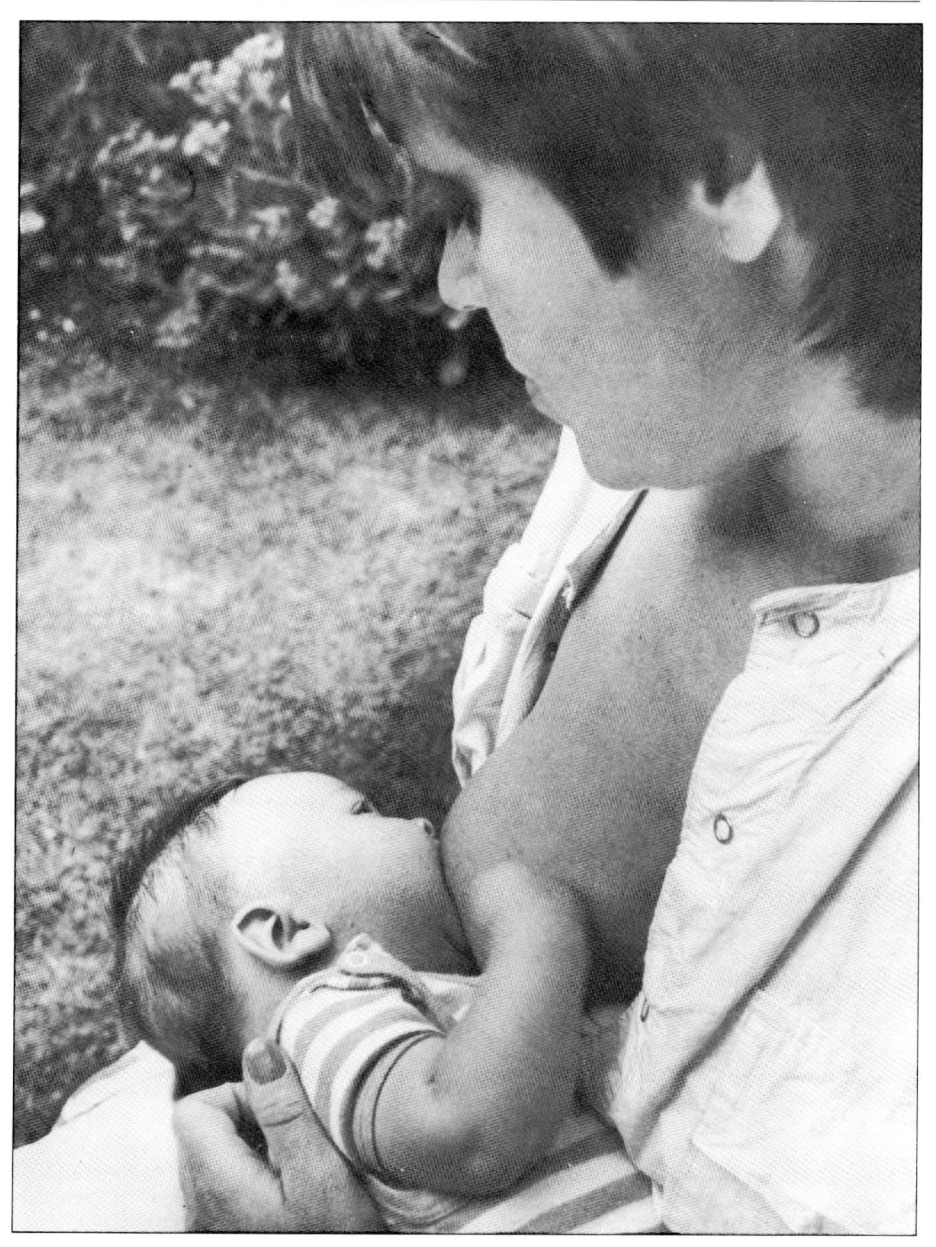

Babies soon learn how to latch on correctly – though you may need a little help at first.

83

LET-DOWN REFLEX

LET-DOWN REFLEX This is an important reflex in *breastfeeding*. It actually allows the milk to come down from the breast to the nipple, and from there it can be squeezed by the baby into his mouth. It's also known as the milk ejection reflex or the draught reflex. When breastfeeding, you have a small amount of milk in the reservoirs behind the nipple, but a hungry baby soon swallows this. To satisfy his hunger and to grow, he needs the richer, fattier milk stored in the milk cells and in the ducts. The milk comes down with the let-down reflex, caused by the hormone oxytocin, produced by the pituitary gland, in response to the baby's sucks. The sensitive nerve endings in the nipple transmit 'instructions' to the pituitary to produce oxytocin which, in turn makes the tiny muscles round the milk cells and ducts contract, squeezing the milk down towards the reservoirs.

The let-down is a highly sensitive reflex, and it can take time to work efficiently. It may mean a few minutes sucking from your baby before he gets it to work, particularly in the early days and weeks. Eventually, however, it may work so well that the milk is let down as soon as your baby touches the nipple – and it can even work as a response to a baby's cry, or even to thoughts about babies! It can be adversely affected by stress, particularly at first, so it's important to be calm and relaxed when you feed. Some women feel a tingling sensation when the let-down works, whereas other women feel nothing.

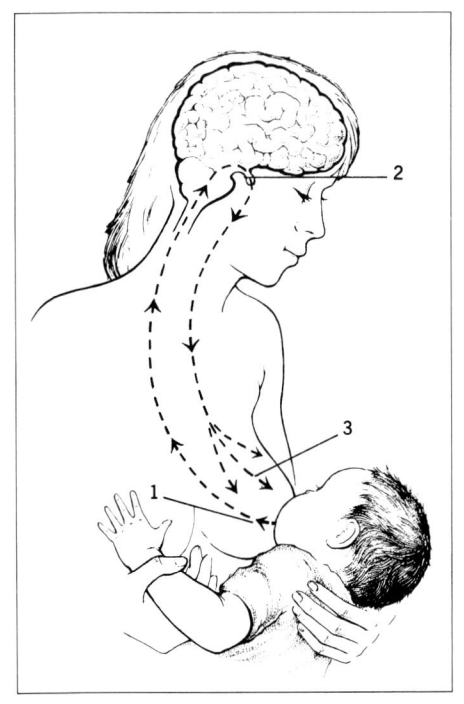

The pressure of the baby's gums on the areola **1** sends signals to the pituitary gland in the brain **2**. This in turn releases the hormone oxytocin which causes the muscle fibres around the milk-storing lobes to contract and force milk into the ducts **3**.

LH Luteinising hormone. This is secreted by the pituitary gland and stimulates the *corpus luteum* to develop after the egg at *ovulation*.

LIE OF BABY IN UTERUS This describes the way the baby is lengthwise in the uterus, towards the end of pregnancy. Normally, the lie is longitudinal, that is, straight up or straight down (though with the legs, arms and chin tucked in). Occasionally, the lie is *transverse* (across the uterus), or oblique (to one side). These positions often correct themselves, and if they don't labour will be obstructed.

LIGHTENING This is the feeling you may get towards the end of pregnancy (usually in the last three to four weeks) when the baby's head drops right down into your pelvis. This lightens the pressure you may have felt against your diaphragm, and it can actually help with any feelings of breathlessness. Mothers having their second or subsequent child don't experience lightening until just before or at the onset of labour (see *engagement of the head*).

LITHOTOMY POSITION

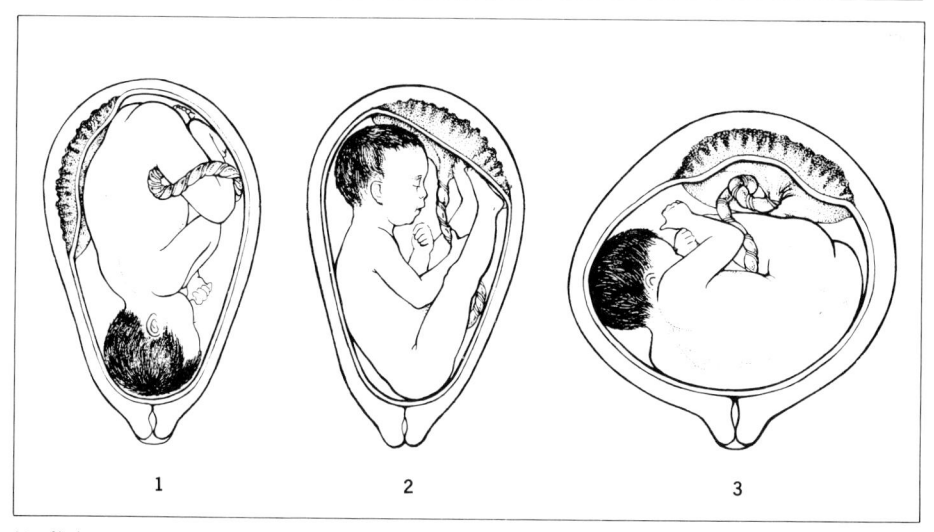

Lie of baby in uterus.
1 Cephalic or head down. This is the most usual form of presentation. **2** Breech. **3** Transverse.

LIGHT-FOR-DATES This describes a baby who is not as big as she should be for the length of time she has been in the uterus (the other terms sometimes used are small-for-dates or dysmature). Light-for-dates babies are often born prematurely, and, as well as problems associated with being born too soon, they are likely to have special problems because of their small size. Some babies are light-for-dates because the placenta hasn't nourished them well enough; some have grown poorly because of some congenital abnormality; very often they are just small, with nothing else wrong at all. However, even a full-term light-for-dates infant may have problems feeding, because she is not quite strong enough to suck with the necessary vigour. Her stomach may only be able to cope with small amounts of milk at any one time, and she may be a sleepy feeder. If your baby is like this, calmness, patience and waking her up for feeds will help.

LINEA NIGRA The dark line you may see during pregnancy on your skin, extending from your pubic area to your navel, and sometimes beyond. It's more noticeable in dark-haired women, and if you're very fair skinned you mightn't notice it at all. This sort of pigmentation can occur elsewhere on the body during pregnancy, and it's due to increased hormonal activity. The linea nigra starts to fade a few weeks after the baby is born, but in some cases it never completely disappears.

LIQUOR See *amniotic fluid*.

LITHOTOMY POSITION One of the standard delivery positions in this country, though rarely used outside Western hospitals. The mother lies flat on her back, her legs raised and bent at the knees. Her legs are supported in lithotomy stirrups, or in a variation, by an attendant at each side. It's been called by the critics the 'stranded beetle position'. From the mother's point of view, and the baby's, it has great disadvantages in a normal labour. However, it *is* necessary for

LOCHIA

forceps deliveries and most doctors in this country prefer it for breech births, too (see *birth position*).

LOCHIA The discharge that comes from your uterus in the days and weeks following birth. You'll need to wear very absorbent sanitary pads to keep yourself clean and comfortable. Tampons are completely out, though, because of the risk of infection, and because the midwife needs to see the lochia when she examines you, to check on the colour and amount. In the first days after the birth the lochia is red, and it consists mainly of blood. The colour then changes through the next days to a sort of pinkish-brown getting paler as time goes on until it's a greenish or creamy colour. When you start getting more active again, it's normal for the lochia to turn red for a few hours, but if you get persistent red lochia, tell your midwife, doctor or health visitor. There's no set time when you expect the lochia to end, and in some women the discharge can last several weeks. If you're breastfeeding you may expect it to end sooner rather than later, as breastfeeding encourages the uterus to contract and thus shed the lochia.

LOW-LYING PLACENTA This is a potentially problematical situation. Normally the placenta places itself in the upper part of the uterus, but occasionally this doesn't happen, and it ends up in the lower segment. When the uterus contracts (as it does all the way through pregnancy, and of course more strongly in labour) the contraction may be strong enough to stretch this part of the uterus and cause some of the placenta to come away slightly from the uterine wall. This causes bleeding, and is obviously dangerous. An *ultrasound* scan will detect just exactly where the placenta is and if it's not too far down, then a normal labour is possible (though some doctors feel this is grounds for induction, so as not to risk a heavy bleed before labour begins). True *placenta praevia* means a *caesarean section* is inevitable.

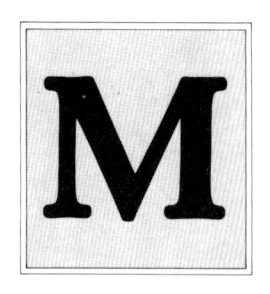

M

MANUAL REMOVAL OF THE PLACENTA This is an emergency treatment, done under epidural or general anaesthetic, when a recently delivered mother has (or risks having) a severe *post-partum haemorrhage* because the placenta hasn't come away from the uterus, and the blood vessels of the uterus have not closed off. The midwife or doctor inserts a hand into the uterus and gently detaches the placenta. Manual removal is sometimes needed if the placenta has become trapped; it may have separated from the uterine wall, but not been able to escape from the uterus because the lower part of the uterus has clamped shut. This is something that occasionally happens after an injection has been given at the *third stage of labour*.

MASSAGE Your partner can massage you in pregnancy for its own sake, or as preparation for massage during labour itself. Massage can help in labour to dissolve tension, encourage relaxed rhythmic breathing and provide warm, emotional support. Many ante-natal classes for couples teach massage techniques with labour in mind, but you can certainly devise your own way of massaging, as different women find different movements helpful. Massage can be anything from the lightest of light surface stroking (often helpful at the base of the spine during contractions), to kneading a muscle and then releasing it (good for releasing tension in the shoulder muscles). There are helpful books around on massage, and some useful chapters in childbirth books.

MASTITIS An infection in the breasts. There are two sorts. The first (sometimes termed superficial mastitis) is a true infection, where a germ has entered the milk (possibly through a hospital-based infection, or perhaps from the baby's nose) and caused the milk to become infected. You may feel aching, tired, hot and cold, with a red sore patch on your breast. The second sort (intramammary mastitis) often follows on from *blocked ducts*. The milk has built up in one part of the breast and has started to leak into the bloodstream. The blood fights the foreign protein in the milk by producing infection-like symptoms, just as in superficial mastitis. You should see a doctor if you suspect you have mastitis, but on no account stop feeding. Sudden cessation of breastfeeding with mastitis can cause a *breast abscess*. If you need to stop offering milk from the affected breast (on doctor's advice), you should continue expressing the milk until you start feeding normally again.

MATERNITY LEAVE If you have been working full-time in the same job for two years at the 11th week before your baby is due, you are probably entitled to maternity leave. This means your job is held open for you for a total of 29 weeks after your baby is born. Some jobs have better arrangements (your job may be held open for longer or you may have an option of returning part-time if that suits you better), whereas other employers are exempt from offering maternity leave for some reason. Part-time workers have to have worked longer with the same employer to claim maternity leave. If you've had previous maternity leave, don't worry; for the purposes of working out the current entitlement, it counts as continuous employment.

You need to let your employer know you intend to return. Tell him in writing 21 days before stopping work that you are coming back at the end of your maternity leave (he may require a signed form from your doctor or midwife to prove your expected date of confinement). Then 21 days before returning, write again, with the date of your return. If your employer writes to you asking you to confirm your intention to return (he cannot do this sooner than 7 weeks after your confinement) you have to reply within 14 days.

To be clear exactly what your rights and entitlements are, speak to your personnel officer, your trade union or to the Department of Employment.

MATERNITY RIGHTS After several years during which women and their employers have almost become used to the machinery of benefits, grants and allowances paid to pregnant women (both working and non-working) and new mothers, all is set to change in 1987 and 1988.

At the time of writing, the changes have not yet been set up – and if and when they are they may only have a short life if a future administration decides to overhaul the system again (hopefully to improve it).

One major change in the new rules means that some pregnant women – those not on supplementary benefit and without a recent work record – will receive no money at all. This group will include girls under 16. The new maternity grant of £75 will be means-tested and only women on supplementary benefit or family income supplement will receive the whole amount.

Working women will be able to apply for Statutory Maternity Pay or state maternity allowance. Statutory Maternity Pay (SMP) will be payable by the employer, and the state maternity allowance will be paid by the Department of Health and Social Security. SMP will be payable for 18 weeks at one or both of two rates and whether you get the lower rate, or a combination of six weeks at the higher rate and 12 weeks at the lower one, depends on the length of time you have worked for the same employer.

Women who don't qualify for SMP but who have paid sufficient National Insurance contributions will get state maternity

MATERNITY WEAR

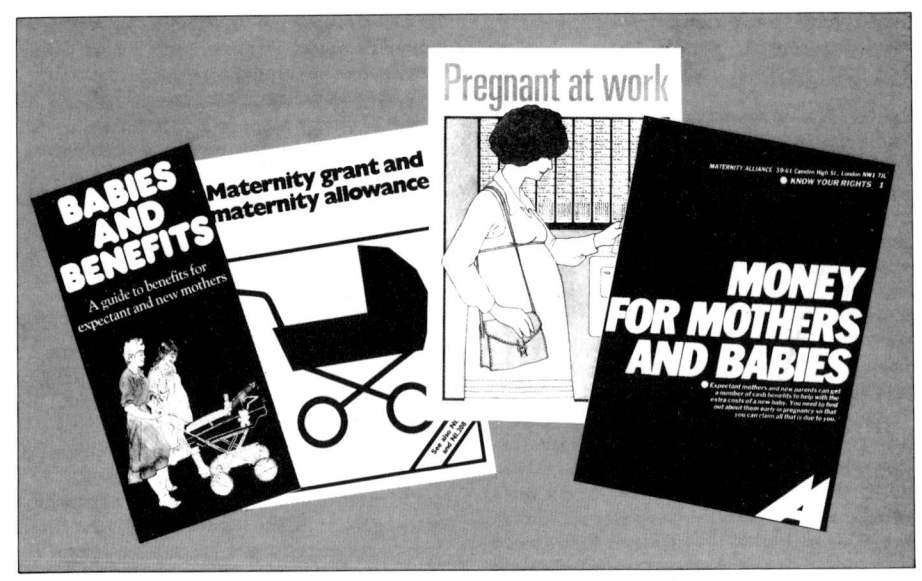

Leaflets available from the DHSS, Health Education Council and Maternity Alliance can help you work out your entitlements.

allowance. This will be less than the lower rate of SMP and is likely to be the same amount as is paid to people entitled to sickness benefit.

This is absolutely the bare bones of it – the full details are much more complex, and the whole system looks no more straightforward than the old one.

Organisations like the Maternity Alliance (see Useful Addresses) and your trades union will give you up-to-date information on your entitlements.

MATERNITY WEAR Most women find they stop being able to fit into some of their normal clothes from the fourth or fifth month of pregnancy, though the looser clothing fashionable these days can mean much of what you already have can double up as maternity wear. You can even wear normal jeans with a loose top for a few extra weeks if you leave the top button undone, the zip unfastened, and keep the whole thing together with a piece of elastic or a belt. When you do start buying maternity clothes look for things you can wear while breastfeeding after the birth (don't expect to be able to leap straight back into jeans as soon as your baby's born). You'll not want them to scream 'pregnant' at you either, because of their styling, if you'd like to wear them later. Dungarees can look great on a lot of pregnant women, though if you get to be pretty big they're not always flattering. Track suits are comfortable too. Choose easy-care fabrics, preferably natural ones so your body can breathe and loose armholes for comfort.

Bras are necessary for most women, though you may be able to carry on wearing your normal pants as they will sit under the bump. Tights can start to be uncomfortable. Even maternity tights develop a roll-over-and-under top once your bump is large. Outsize tights worn back to front (so the bit that's meant to go over large ladies' behinds goes over your tum) can be just as good, and are probably cheaper. Support stockings – though no longer tights – are available at the chemist on prescription. If you need a coat, a tent-shape, lightweight raincoat (worn with layers of woollies underneath if it's cold) is better than a proper maternity coat (which will look huge and feel uncomfortably heavy both during and after pregnancy).

Good sources of maternity wear include Indian shops that sell soft floaty cotton frocks, second-hand shops and jumble sales. If you know someone who's been pregnant recently, ask if you can borrow some maternity clothes. However, it's good for your morale to buy one or two things that you feel you look really good in.

MECONIUM This is the first substance passed from the bowels of a newborn. In the first days it's greenish black, and then it gradually changes colour until the bowel passes the normal, yellow-coloured soft motions of a breastfed baby. Bottle-fed babies' stools are paler and firmer. The midwife will ask you if your baby has passed meconium. When he does, it's a good sign that there's no intestinal or rectal blockage.

MEDICAL HISTORY You will be asked about your medical background when you're pregnant as it can have a bearing on your health during pregnancy and afterwards. You'll need to say if you've had any serious illnesses, whether you're on medication, if you have a heart condition, for example. Previous pregnancies and their outcome will be noted, too (see *booking appointment*).

MEMBRANES Two thin tissues enclosing the fetus and the amniotic fluid in the uterus, forming the 'bag' of the bag of waters (see *amniotic sac*).

MIDWIFE A midwife is usually, though not always, a nurse who has done special training on top of her general and other nursing qualifications. A few midwives have done a 'direct entry' course without having done nursing first. Either way, she is highly qualified to understand and where necessary help with the processes of normal pregnancy and labour. The word midwife literally means 'with woman' and the tradition of women helping other women have their babies is a long and admirable one, and one that's common to most cultures and periods of history. These days, midwives generally work in hospital, or within the community as *community midwives*. The community midwife looks after women having their babies at home; she works in GP or health centre ante-natal clinics, and health centre classes, and she visits women with new babies after they have been discharged from hospital. In hospital, you will see hospital midwives in the ante-natal clinic and in ante-natal classes, during the birth itself and afterwards on the post-natal wards.

Midwives are also trained in the care of young babies and of newly delivered mothers, and they will help you with breastfeeding.

In one or two hospitals, you may meet a male midwife, though they are a rare breed (until recently, training and employment restrictions applied). If you'd feel happiest with a female midwife, though, don't hesitate to say so.

MILK BANKS Many hospitals with special care baby units run a milk bank, where breast milk is stored to be given later to sick or pre-term babies. The bank is kept stocked by volunteer mothers, who collect their own 'spare' breast milk (perhaps by expressing, perhaps by collecting the 'drip' milk that may leak from their breasts). Local branches of organisations such as the National Childbirth Trust usually undertake to run the milk bank collection procedure, and hospital staff apply certain standards to the milk they accept (though these standards differ from hospital to hospital), and donors will be checked for various health factors.

If your own baby needs special care, and you are unable to feed him for some reason, ask if he can be given breast milk from the milk bank, as for many sick and pre-term babies this can be better than formula milk.

MISCARRIAGE

MISCARRIAGE The loss of a baby before 28 weeks gestation. Miscarriage is commonest in the first 12 weeks of pregnancy. Estimates vary as to the number of pregnancies that end in miscarriage, it could be as high as one in five. Very early miscarriages can happen before the woman even knows she is pregnant – she may have what appears to be a heavy period, possibly accompanied by some pain or discomfort. Miscarriage is usually preceded by bleeding from the vagina and cramp-like pains. You need to contact a doctor if this happens to you.

The causes of miscarriage aren't always known. In many cases however it's thought that miscarriage is 'nature's way' of disposing of a less-than-perfect conception. When miscarried fetuses are studied, it's often found that there are chromosomal abnormalities. In other cases the fertilised egg hasn't even begun to develop normally, and miscarriage is the inevitable outcome. When miscarriage happens later in pregnancy, it may be because the mother's cervix has failed to stay closed (*incompetent cervix*) and the baby is miscarried as the mother goes into what is, in effect, very early labour. This condition can be dealt with by means of a *Shirodkar stitch* in the cervix.

After a miscarriage, you may be advised to have a D & C, to make sure your uterus is clear of the pregnancy. Always ask the doctor for his opinion on why you miscarried; even if he can't be sure why, you need to be able to discuss it.

The vast majority of women who miscarry go on to have a subsequent, normal, pregnancy. Even the few who suffer *recurrent abortion* can often be helped. Nevertheless, miscarriage can be deeply distressing and traumatic to both mother and father, and there's no reason to feel odd or freakish if you need to grieve. Counselling and emotional support can help (see *blighted ovum, hydatidiform mole*, Useful Addresses).

MONITOR See *fetal monitor*.

MONTGOMERY'S TUBERCLES These are the small nodules that appear round the nipple in early pregnancy. Their function is to secrete a sort of fluid that keeps the nipples soft. They don't go away completely between pregnancies, but in a first-time mother they can be taken as a sign of pregnancy.

MORNING SICKNESS See *sickness*.

MOULDING Because a new baby's skull bones are not yet fused together, his head is temporarily shaped during birth by his descent down the birth canal – the bones actually slide over one another. This shaping is known as moulding; it soon disappears (see *fontanelle, head of baby*).

MOVEMENT IN LABOUR Moving around is becoming recognised as the sensible thing to do during a normal labour. Fewer and fewer hospitals are insisting on confining you to bed as soon as they have admitted you. Freedom to experiment with different positions during contractions, and the chance to remain upright, can help the progress of labour and reduce the need for pain-relieving drugs.

MUCUS EXTRACTION In many hospitals, babies are routinely 'sucked out' by the midwife after birth. This process is called mucus extraction, and it takes away any mucus that may be blocking the baby's airways and preventing him from breathing properly. Basically, it involves a fine rubber tube being placed in the baby's nose and mouth and although the operation is quick and simple in experienced hands, and obviously life-saving in some instances, its routine application is certainly questionable. A baby who is already breathing normally (and this is usually simple for a midwife to assess) hardly needs what must be something of an uncomfortable procedure. Discuss this with your ante-natal clinic, and ask their opinion. If you feel strongly that a healthy

MULTIPLE PREGNANCY

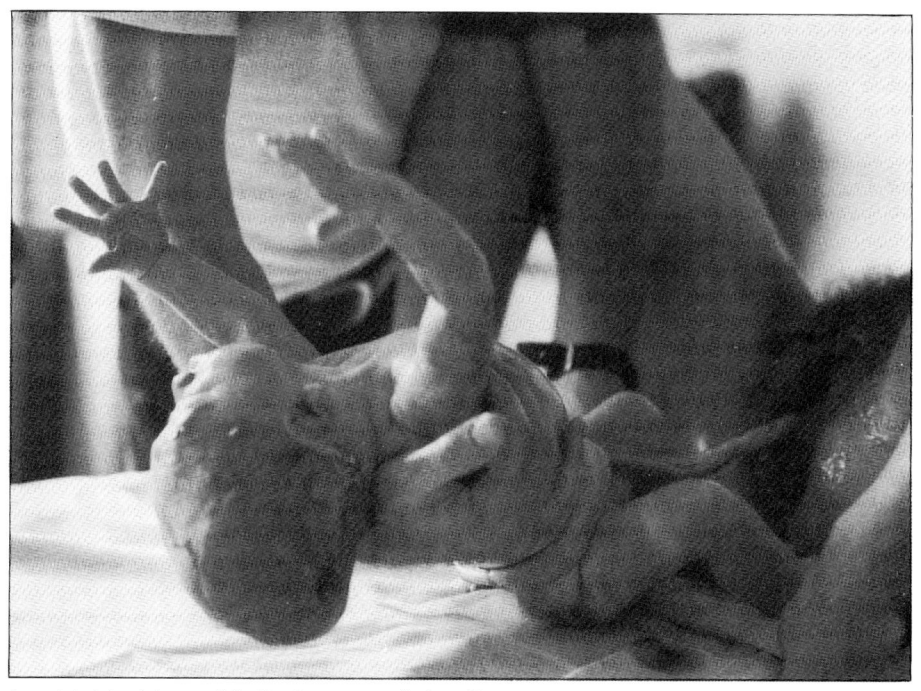

A new baby's head shows a distinctive shape as a result of moulding.

baby shouldn't be subjected to mucus extraction, then say so.

MUCUS PLUG See *show*.

MULTIGRAVIDA A woman who has been pregnant more than once.

MULTIPARA A woman who has previously given birth more than once.

MULTIPLE PREGNANCY Any pregnancy where more than one baby is expected (see *twins, triplets*).

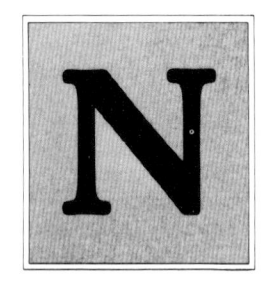

N.A.D. An abbreviation of the phrase 'nothing abnormal discovered'. It's often written by doctors and midwives on your notes in columns where the result of (for example) urine testing is recorded. It really means 'okay'.

NAPPIES In this country, we cling to our traditional terry towelling squares for our babies, though the heavily advertised disposable nappies are making great inroads into the market. Disposables are convenient and much more absorbent than they used to be. Even with automatic washing machines terries are a chore to wash, and a nightmare to dry if you have neither a tumble dryer nor washing line. But large packets of disposables are bulky to bring back from the shops (although you can order in bulk with free delivery from some suppliers) and not all types are satisfactorily disposable. Ecologically speaking, terries win on points as they can be washed (endlessly . . .) to use again and again, and they last through at least two children.

Surprisingly, there's not a lot to choose between the two methods on price, because although, nappy-by-nappy, disposables are more costly, terries need electricity to heat the water in the washing machine, sterilising powder to soak them in beforehand, washing powder, liners, plastic pants and pins and this all brings the total closer than you'd think. Most parents these days seem to be voting with their feet in this debate: they're buying terries for use in the first months when you can plough your way through six to ten nappies a day, and switching to disposables for outings and holidays, and for when their babies are toddling.

NAPPY CHANGING A midwife will show you how to change your baby's nappy, and you'll get better at it with plenty of practice. While your baby's small, you'll need to change him about as often as you feed him; however, if he feeds little and often over a long period of time, don't take that rule too literally, or you'll not have time to do anything else. Double nappies, or a very absorbent sort of disposable can sometimes rule out the need for night time changing, too. A small baby's bottom needs to be washed at every nappy change, and possibly creamed or oiled, to prevent nappy rash.

NATURAL CHILDBIRTH A term that's often used, but the user and the listener sometimes have different ideas on its definition. Basically, it should mean childbirth allowed to proceed without any medical help or interference in the form of drugs or machinery. But few people would argue that women should be able to give birth literally on their own, without a midwife to check on their progress and the health and safety of their baby, although if we take the word 'natural' literally, it could actually mean that! Other definitions mean something to do with just not having any pharmacological pain-relief, although a woman might be attached to a monitor, and be made to stay in bed throughout her labour. In the past, women have set out to have natural births, and because everything has not proceeded normally, have ended up with a caesarean section or forceps, and have been disappointed because this meant the birth wasn't 'natural', and was somehow sub-standard.

I prefer the newer term *'active birth'*. Implicit in it is the idea that women can and should

NAPPY CHANGING

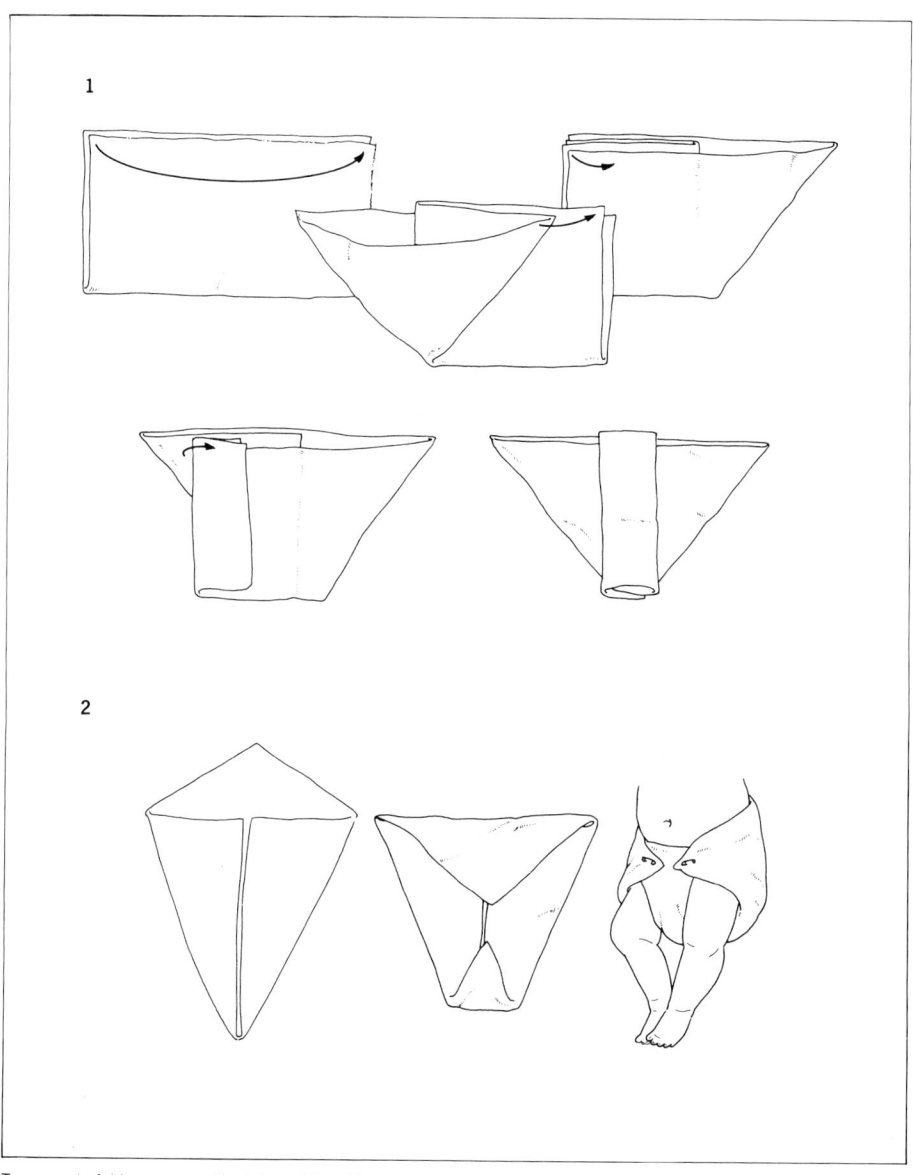

Two ways to fold a nappy are the 'origami' **1** and the 'kite' **2** method.
1 This gives a neat fit, and good absorbency at the front.
2 This is adjustable in size as the upper and lower points of the kite shape can be brought closer together to give a smaller nappy when needed.

give birth with confidence, and without unnecessary medical procedures that might hamper this. But the emphasis in active birth is not on the 'naturalness' of the event, but on the involvement and control of the woman. So, it would be perfectly possible to have an active birth that ended in forceps, or caesarean section for sound obstetric reasons, but because the woman would be aware that the forceps or section were needed for her safety and that of the baby, the birth could not then suddenly become 'inactive'. In any case, the opposite of 'active' doesn't have the perjorative tone of the word 'unnatural'!

NAUSEA The sort of sick feeling you can get at any time, but particularly in the first three months, of pregnancy (see *sickness, vomiting*).

NAVEL The other word for the umbilicus. It's the scar left on your skin in the middle of your abdomen which marks the spot where the umbilical cord was.

NEURAL TUBE DEFECTS These are the conditions *spina bifida* and *anencephaly*.

NIPPLE SHIELD This can be a help during breastfeeding if the nipples have become sore or cracked, or where the baby is having difficulty in *latching on* to a very *flat* or *inverted* nipple, but it shouldn't be used for too long or your baby might get rather too accustomed to it, and find it difficult to get used to sucking directly from the nipple itself. Long-term use might be needed though if your nipples remain flat or inverted. Some nipple shields are made of rubber; others have a glass or polycarbonate-type base attached to a rubber bottle teat. Both these work in the same way, by fitting over the nipple while the baby sucks milk through a hole or holes in the end. You need to sterilise the shield between feeds, of course. It's been shown that thin latex shields reduce the milk flow less that other types, so this sort could be the first one to try if you need a shield.

NOTES These are the sheets of information about you and your pregnancy, and they include the results of any tests you may have had, correspondence from your GP, and a record of your ante-natal visits. Your notes will pop up in the cubicle at the ante-natal clinic while you wait for your check-up, and the doctor or midwife will look at them and record his or her own observations on them. If you have shared ante-natal care with your GP, you will have a *co-operation card* which is a sort of mini-version of your hospital notes. You keep your co-op card yourself, but on the front of your notes you may see a stern warning about not reading them, or about them being the property of the hospital. It seems daft that we therefore feel guilty about sneaking a peep at them ourselves. It means that if we see something we don't understand in our own notes, we daren't even ask about it because we aren't supposed to be reading them anyway! Ideally every mother should make a point of looking at her notes occasionally, and asking about them. After all, it's your body! One other point: if you have any 'special requests' about the way you want to have your baby, get the doctor or midwife to write them up in your notes. That way, the midwife who admits you in labour has a sort of official sanction to do something (or not do something) that may be different from the usual hospital routine.

baby can cause contractions you feel in your back. In a few cases, the head doesn't turn properly and forceps are needed to complete the delivery. Sometimes, the delivery is a *face presentation* (the baby is born face first) or a *brow presentation*. The main disadvantage with posterior positions is that they can make labour longer and more uncomfortable, though this is by no means inevitable.

OCCIPUT *(óx-i-put)* The back of a baby's head.

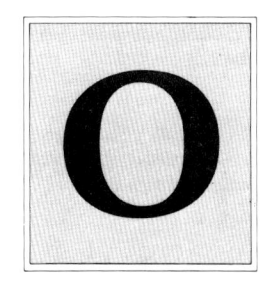

OBSERVATIONS IN LABOUR The routine observations the midwife will make when you're in labour will include regular pulse and blood pressure checks, a four-hourly (at least) internal examination to see whether the cervix is dilating as it should be, and to check the descent of the baby's head, a check on the strength and length of your contractions (done by placing a hand in your uterus during a contraction). The baby's heart will be listened to and the rate noted (heart rate and contractions can both be recorded electronically and continuously with a *fetal monitor*). In addition, the urine you pass during labour will be tested routinely for *ketones*.

OBSTETRICIAN A doctor who specialises in and who has professional qualifications in pregnancy, labour, birth and the puerperium (the period after birth). Many obstetricians will also be gynaecologists.

OCCIPITO POSTERIOR *(ox-í-pitto posterior)* This describes one way the baby can be positioned in the uterus. His back is towards your back. It's not ideal because in this position he can't get well-flexed. He doesn't have the space to tuck his chin and his legs in and his head won't engage quite so well. He can be right occipito posterior with his back to the right of the middle of yours (ROP), or left occipito posterior (LOP). Labour with an OP

OEDEMA Fluid retention in the tissues of the body causing puffiness or swelling, not uncommon in pregnancy. You can get it round your ankles, fingers, wrists, face. Plenty of rest and lying with your feet up can help. In most cases it's a nuisance that has to be put up with, and it's something that disappears anyway after delivery. If it's combined with high blood pressure, however, it can be a sign of *pre-eclampsia*, so any excessive or sudden swelling should be reported to your doctor or midwife (see *ankles, swollen*).

OESTRiOL *(eestriol)* A hormone secreted by the placenta, excreted in the urine and present in the blood of a pregnant woman.

OESTRIOL TESTS Tests carried out by a hospital to estimate the amount of the hormone oestriol being secreted by the placenta during pregnancy. This can give an indication of whether the placenta is working efficiently or not, and blood samples and/or urine collections are tested for oestriol in late pregnancy especially to assess the growth rate of the fetus. The main problem with 'oestriols' is that the tests aren't very accurate: there is such a wide variation in what's normal, the tests have to be repeated over a period of time to get the best possible individual result. Women with a low oestriol count have given birth to perfectly normal-sized babies. Others with good oestriols have had light-for-dates

OESTROGENS

babies. The main hazard therefore is that babies may be induced unnecessarily (because it's thought the placenta is about to stop functioning efficiently), or that babies are allowed to go to term and beyond when they would be better off being born. It's for these reasons that many obstetricians like to ask the mother to keep a *kick chart* instead, or to combine a kick chart with oestriols. In any case, if there's no particular reason to suspect a placental insufficiency, you may not have any oestriol tests done.

OESTROGENS *(eestrojens)* A group of sex hormones that causes breasts to develop at puberty and which initiate the onset of menstruation. During pregnancy, oestrogens help to prepare the breasts for lactation and they cause the lining of the womb to become thicker.

OLD WIVES' TALES There's no doubt that a lot of old wives' tales about pregnancy and birth are at least misleading and at worst dangerously false. But don't dismiss everything your granny tells you. Women can pass on accumulated and inherited experience where motherhood is concerned, and that shared knowledge and wisdom can be lovingly meant and supportive to you.

OPERCULUM The plug of mucus which seals the cervix throughout pregnancy. It's loosened towards the start of labour and is expelled as a sort of pinkish streaky blob (though you might not, in fact, notice it), called the *show*.

ORGASM A sexual climax. When the man ejaculates, he experiences orgasm as well. Therefore, with him, conception is physiologically linked with orgasm. However, a woman doesn't need to have an orgasm in order to conceive. *Intercourse* – including orgasm – is perfectly safe for both men and women during pregnancy (unless your doctor advises otherwise), as are all forms of sexual activity (bar blowing air into the vagina, which could lead to an embolism). It is claimed that orgasm is one way of getting an overdue labour started.

OS (OF THE CERVIX) The opening in the *cervix*, normally closed during pregnancy with a plug of mucus (see *operculum*).

OVULATION The term used to describe the release of a ripened egg (ovum) from the ovary, for possible fertilisation. Ovulation occurs about 14 days before the next menstrual period would normally be expected (see *conception*).

OXYGEN A gas essential to life. The fetus gets his oxygen supply through his blood, which is oxygenated when it reaches the placenta through the umbilical cord. It then goes back again to his body, and circulates, taking oxygen to all parts of the body. When he is born, he will take his oxygen from the air by breathing it in. A baby is in danger if he has breathing difficulties and can't take in sufficient oxygen; this can cause brain damage. Tiny or sick babies may need help with their breathing, and be given extra oxygen. The amount given is precisely regulated these days, as too much oxygen can cause the tragedy of blindness.

OXYTOCIN A hormone produced in the pituitary gland responsible for making the uterus contract. It's now produced synthetically (and known as syntocinon) and used in a solution to induce or accelerate labour. Ocytocin (the natural sort) is also vital in breastfeeding as it is this hormone that produces the *let-down reflex* to cause the milk to be made available to the baby (see *acceleration, induction*).

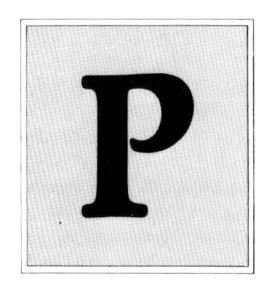

PAIN IN LABOUR This is quite an issue! It's easy to caricature opposing viewpoints as the debate has become quite heated recently. At one extreme, it appears a healthy woman should approach childbirth confidently, with the opportunity to give birth with no unnecessary medical interference, and with loving support from her partner and the midwife. In this way, she is unlikely to experience much pain. In fact, 'strong contractions' (rather than 'pain') can be welcomed, and even compared to the sexual excitement of making love. At the other extreme we have the approach advocated by American comedienne Joan Rivers, whose ideal birth is to be 'knocked out at the first twinge and wake up in the hairdresser's'! Childbirth is an ordeal, they say, and women should grab the chance of effective pain relief, dissociating themselves from the 'lentil eating earth mothers' scoffed at by Polly Toynbee (*Guardian*, 1986), who are the campaigners for 'natural childbirth'.

If there's any sort of general truth to be gleaned, it is that all of us are different, and our pain thresholds differ, too. There is no doubt that a frightened, confused and distressed mother is more likely to experience her labour contractions as unbearably painful, and a confident, happy one is more likely to have a relaxed, positive labour experience, although she may still experience her contractions as painful. At present, truly painfree labour without an *epidural* is a rarity, though it could become less rare as women are given the freedom to give birth in the way they want to. I feel, though, that to be realistic, we should expect some pain in labour. For most, however, the pain isn't continuous. Even the most painful contractions (usually at the end of the first stage) come and go, with a welcome respite between them. If you've ever had painful periods, the pain may remind you of that although more intense. Some women report that it's like a tightening belt; others say it's like a backache.

Your experience of pain does not have to prevent your experience of birth from being a happy, joyful and positive one. The energy and effort you put into labour can be part of the wonderful sense of achievement you feel at creating and bringing forth a new, loved person. However, the important factor in all this is that women wanted to be treated with respect and courtesy in labour, and to have their wishes about pain relief acknowledged, and where possible, acted upon. There should be effective pain relief available at all times for all who want it – with no pressure put on those who don't. There's no room for guilt at having had pain relief, nor smugness at having done without.

PAIN RELIEF (IN LABOUR) See *active birth, breathing in labour, entonox, epidural anaesthesia, pethidine, psychoprophylaxis, relaxation, TNS*.

PALPATION Examination by touching. At the ante-natal clinic a midwife or doctor will use her palms and her fingers to gently press on your abdomen, in order to assess the size of the uterus and the size and position of the baby.

PANTING IN LABOUR This is sometimes used as part of the breathing techniques taught in ante-natal classes, and many midwives encourage their mothers to use it in labour in the second stage. Its basic function is to suspend activity for a short time, to prevent a mother *bearing down*, so that the baby's head can be born slowly and gently.

PARENTCRAFT

PARENTCRAFT Most ante-natal classes have at least some of their curriculum devoted to talking about parentcraft – the practical day-to-day care of a new baby, and discussions on how 'life after birth' will change. When given in a non-dogmatic way, parentcraft can be helpful, particularly for first-time parents with no experience of babies before. National Health Service classes in particular are sometimes criticised for an approach that borders on the rigid, however: parentcraft becomes a set of rules and routines about bathing, feeding and shopping lists of baby equipment. Strict ideas these days are out-of-step with most modern mother's needs, and apart from basic common sense about warmth, safety and hygiene, there aren't (or shouldn't be) any rigid rules about baby care.

PATERNITY LEAVE Not usually given in this country, though hopefully this will change one day. Some enlightened employers give as much as a fortnight's paid leave to new fathers; other fathers can actually lose pay by being with their partners in labour. Whether or not you get formal paternity leave, it's worth trying to take some sort of time off (perhaps some annual holiday) to get used to life as a family.

PELVIC FLOOR EXERCISES The pelvic floor is formed of strong sheets of muscle that support and enclose the pelvic organs (in the woman, these are the uterus, fallopian tubes, ovaries, bladder and rectum, though of course men have a pelvic floor too). The pelvic floor exercises you may be taught to do in your ante-natal classes (and which should be done before and after delivery) strengthen these muscles and improve their tone. The main exercise is very simple to do, and is amazingly effective in curing any feeling of 'laxness' in the pelvic floor you may get after the birth. It involves contracting and releasing the muscles surrounding the urethra, vagina and anus (it helps to imagine them as a figure of eight). One way of seeing how the exercise works is to stop and start the flow of urine a few times as you pass water, by contracting the muscles and releasing them.

PERI-NATAL The time from before delivery to seven days after.

PERI-NATAL DEATH The death of a baby before, during or in the week after birth. The peri-natal mortality rate considers all stillbirths and neo-natal deaths and considers them as a figure per 1000 births.

PERINEUM The area between the vagina and the anus. During childbirth it becomes flattened out and stretched by the baby's head, and the skin becomes very thin. It's this area that's cut when an *episiotomy* is done. It can also tear during delivery.

PESSARIES Objects containing some sort of drug inserted into the vagina. *Prostaglandin* pessaries can be used to induce labour. Other sorts may be prescribed, during pregnancy or otherwise, for vaginal infection (see *induction*).

PETHIDINE Pethidine is a very commonly given drug to help with the pain during labour. Its main effects are to relax you, and to distance you slightly from everything, including the pain you have been feeling. For some women it's very effective. Others dislike the feeling of lack of control it can give. It can make you sleepy, so you sleep between contractions and then wake up with a jolt at the very height of the next one. If you are keen on breathing techniques in labour, then pethidine is not likely to enhance your ability to concentrate on them. Having said that, some women find it's helpful to have the edge of consciousness blurred in this way.

Pethidine is usually given by injection, and the effects take about 15 or 20 minutes to work. If you really aren't sure whether you'll appreciate the effects, you could ask for half a

PLACENTA PRAEVIA

dose to start off with (the standard first dose is often 100 or 150 mg though practices vary). It's important that pethidine isn't given too soon before the end of labour as it can depress a new baby's breathing. The baby is also born reluctant to feed and very sleepy, sometimes for several days. To counteract this, some maternity units inject a pethidine antidote (into you, or into the baby after birth) but its effects are sometimes limited.

PHANTOM PREGNANCY See *false pregnancy*.

PHENYLKETONURIA Known as PKU, this is a rare metabolic disorder detected in a new baby by a simple blood test (see *Guthrie test*).

PILES Varicose veins of the anus, also termed haemorrhoids. Often excruciatingly painful, so do all you can to avoid getting one. Make sure you avoid *constipation*, which predisposes to piles. Special creams (from the doctor) can bring relief, and you will probably find that the pile (or piles) disappear or go down after pregnancy.

THE PILL If you've been taking the contraceptive pill and then find you're pregnant, stop taking it. Some experts believe it's sensible to come off the pill and wait for one natural period before trying to conceive; others say wait at least three months (use other contraceptive methods instead during this time). Waiting a few months helps the pregnancy to be dated more accurately, and gives your body a chance to get back to normal hormonal balance. It could also have advantages in allowing your system to make up certain vitamin and mineral deficiencies that are thought to occur with the pill. After giving birth, discuss your contraceptive method with the *family planning* clinic or your doctor. If you're breastfeeding you'll be advised either to avoid the pill or to use the progestogen-only pill which is thought to have no effect on the milk supply, but you may of course wish to think about other methods instead.

PLACENTA The afterbirth, present and fully functioning from the 14th week of pregnancy, is absolutely vital to your baby's growth and survival. It's more or less circular in shape, and on one side it is attached to the wall of the uterus. The *umbilical cord* joins the baby to the placenta, and acts as a two-way link. The placenta is a sort of outpost of your baby's blood circulation and of your own. It passes nutrients (from your blood) into the baby's bloodstream (though your own blood system and your baby's are kept separate). Waste products from the baby also reach the placenta, cross it and thus get passed back to you for your body to deal with. The placenta also acts as a sieve, preventing certain harmful organisms and illnesses from reaching your baby.

After your baby's born the umbilical cord is cut and the placenta is delivered with one or two contractions (if, as is usual, you have been given an injection of hormone to make the uterus expel the placenta as quickly as this). The midwife examines the placenta, mainly to check that it's intact and that the membranes are present, as any part of the placenta left in the uterus can lead to *post-partum haemorrhage* (see *third stage of labour*).

PLACENTA PRAEVIA *(placenta pree-via)* A placenta so low in the uterus that the baby is above it, is termed placenta praevia. It may lie over the cervix, partially or completely blocking the baby's exit. The danger with placenta praevia is severe bleeding, as a result of the placenta breaking away from the uterus. To avoid this, all women with a diagnosed placenta praevia are delivered by caesarean section, whenever possible before they go into spontaneous labour. Placenta praevia is diagnosed by ultrasound and this is done if a woman is admitted to hospital in late pregnancy with bleeding. She may be advised to rest or stay in bed for the rest of her

PLACENTAL ABRUPTION

1 Partial placenta praevia.

2 Full placenta praevia.

PLACENTAL INSUFFICIENCY This describes the condition where the placenta isn't doing the job it needs to, to make sure the baby grows well. The causes of it aren't entirely understood, but poor health and an inadequate diet seem to increase the risk. It can also be caused by severe *pre-eclampsia*, consistently and seriously high *blood pressure*; *smoking* also reduces the effectiveness of the placenta. In most cases, the baby is born *light-for-dates*. In severe cases the result is a stillbirth.

POLYHYDRAMNIOS An excess of *amniotic fluid*. This can cause your uterus to expand greatly to hold it all, and one of the signs of polyhydramnios is a womb that's far larger than dates would indicate. The condition can be associated with complications (it may, for instance, be caused by a malformed baby unable to swallow amniotic fluid), or diabetes. In other cases, there appears to be no cause at all and a normal, healthy baby is born.

POSITIONS FOR FIRST STAGE During the first stage of labour, most women are more comfortable if they keep moving around, being just as mobile as they feel they want to be. If you go into labour at night, your very early contractions may be mild enough to let you sleep and you should do this, if you can, to conserve your energy. Sleep eventually becomes impossible, however, once things start getting going, and if you experiment with different positions – kneeling, leaning against a chair, lying on your side, propped up with cushions, squatting, and so on – you'll find what suits you best at any given time. If you are having a home birth or if you stay at home for much of the first stage of labour, you'll probably have lots of chairs, stools and pillows to change position with. Hospitals these days are on the whole less likely to insist in confining you to bed for the whole of your labour, but the use of most types of *fetal monitor* mean you have to remain fairly immobile (this is one of the major disadvantages of the monitor, in fact). You

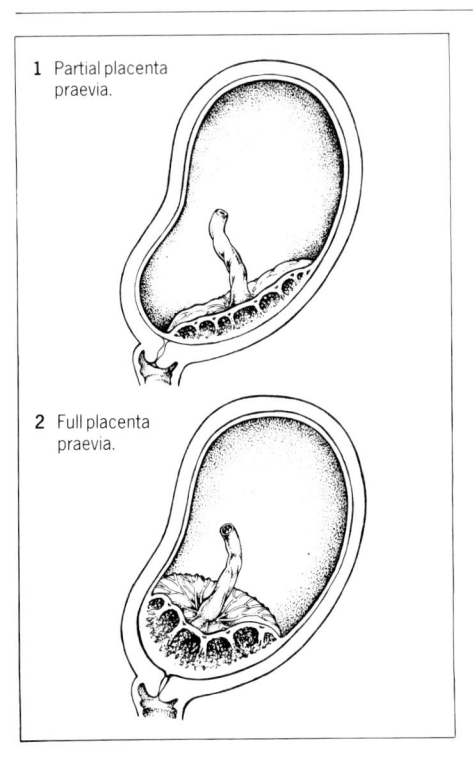

pregnancy (and she may be admitted to hospital) until she gets to around 37 or 38 weeks, when she'll have a caesarean section.

PLACENTAL ABRUPTION (ABRUPTO PLACENTAE) This can happen in late pregnancy if the placenta starts to come away from the wall of the uterus, and the first sign is almost always bleeding from the vagina, possibly with pain. The cause isn't usually known, as the placenta may well be in a normal position in the uterus (as opposed to *placenta praevia*). When the condition is mild – if the bleeding stops and the blood loss hasn't been great – there may be no treatment required. When there has been a lot of blood lost, however, there could be a need for a blood transfusion and emergency delivery of the baby, possibly by caesarean section.

POST-NATAL BLUES

will have to remain lying down with an *epidural* and reasonably still with a *drip* (see *birth positions*).

POSITIONS FOR SECOND STAGE See *birth positions*.

POSTERIOR PRESENTATION See *occipito posterior*.

POST-MATURE (POST-TERM) Some babies who have been in the uterus for 42 weeks or more show some obvious signs of the condition known as post-maturity. These signs are a cracked and peeling skin, and thinnish body, and unless he is ill, the post-term baby will be hungry. This is because he has been born beyond the ideal time and the placenta has deteriorated. Breathing problems and other illnesses aren't uncommon in post-term babies so post-maturity is definitely undesirable – and it's something doctors aim to avoid by *induction* at the right time, before post-maturity develops.

POST-NATAL After the birth.

POST-NATAL BLUES This should really only refer to the emotional low many women experience in the days of the first week or so after delivery. In the popular press, however, it's sometimes used as a general term to include true *post-natal depression*. The blues – sometimes known as third (or fourth) day blues – could be a mixture of the hormonal action causing the milk to come in, together with a come-down after the tremendous

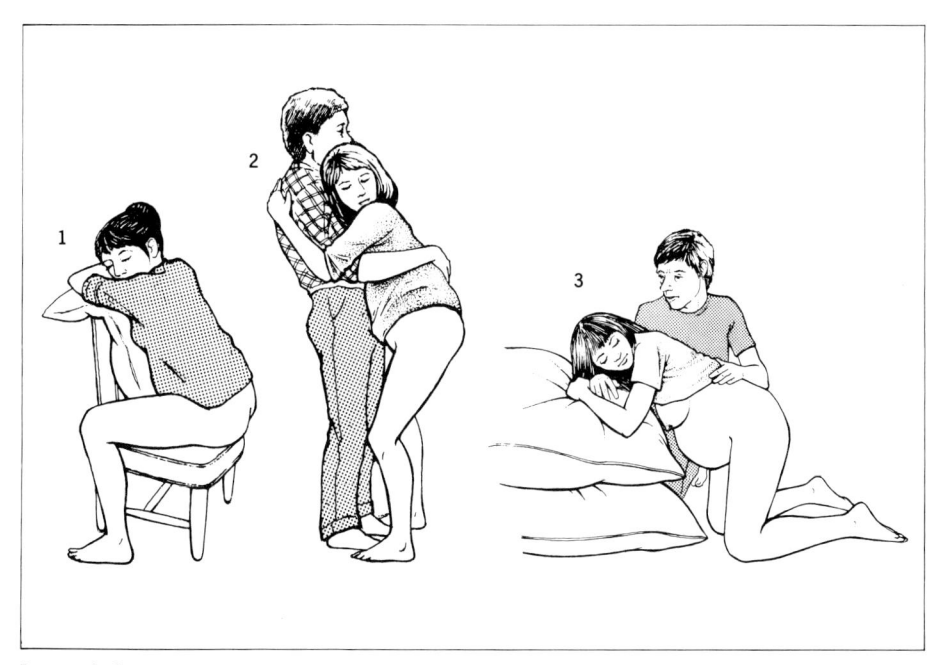

Positions for first stage.
1 Leaning on a chair. **2** Standing and supported by your partner. **3** Propped up on cushions.

POST-NATAL DEPRESSION

elation of giving birth. Whatever it is, post-natal ward staff are well-used to the sight of grown women weeping over small upsets. The emotions are real at the time, but you usually get over them quickly. Even so, new motherhood is often a tearful time, when new responses are engendered, and new feelings aroused. There can come a time for some women, though when the odd bout of tearfulness is only part of a deeper, more pervasive feeling of sadness, inadequacy and out-of-touchness. This, then, could be post-natal depression and medical advice should be sought.

POST-NATAL DEPRESSION There seems to be no truly accurate figures or percentages on post-natal depression, but one thing is clear: it happens more often than we used to think. One estimate is that about one mother in ten suffers from it, though even this glosses over the fact that some women are fine after a few months, whereas others suffer for years. Post-natal depression can take many forms. At its most severe, and obvious, it's a form of psychosis, possibly needing hospitalisation and lengthy after-care. The mother cannot function normally, and she may have delusions about who she is, where she is and who her baby is. Much more commonly, post-natal depression emerges gradually. It may appear in the form of a great sadness, feelings of inadequacy, tremendous fatigue and lethargy, a sensation of living on a different plane to other people, irrational fears. Any or all of these symptoms are typical. Lots of mothers struggle on through them, only breaking down in tears when they are alone, and presenting a 'normal' face to the world, even to their husbands. The babies of mothers with PND are often perfectly well-cared for, and to the outsider there may be no clues anything is wrong.

What should be shouted from the rooftops is that PND is curable; in almost every case, with the right treatment, sympathy and love, a woman can return to her 'real' self, though the road back may be hard. GPs and health visitors are much more clued-up than they were about the symptoms; research into various forms of treatment continues, and self-help and support groups abound. The three main schools of thought about PND are: (1) that it is almost entirely due to the isolation and social disorientation of new mothers and the lack of support they get from those around them, plus, possibly bad labour experiences. It has its roots in women's experience of the world, and in their conditioning. Friends, love and contact can help; (2) that it is a result of hormone imbalances that can be corrected by the right sort of hormone therapy, often given in the form of injections; (3) that it is just another form of depression, curable by the varying approaches of psychotherapy, psychiatry and the judicious prescribing of anti-depressant drugs. There is no doubt that each school of thought can help certain people. The important thing, if PND happens to you, is to admit it – and seek help (see Useful Addresses).

POST-NATAL EXAMINATION This usually takes place six or seven weeks after you've had your baby. It's done either at the hospital, or by your GP or community midwife. You'll be given a *vaginal examination* (and you may have a cervical smear test done at the same time), and the vagina, perineum or cervix will be checked for healing, especially if you've had stitches. The size of your uterus will be felt (it should be down to a non-pregnant size and shape, though it will always be softer than it was before you were pregnant). You may be asked to bring a specimen of urine for testing and you're likely to have your blood pressure checked, too. You should also be asked if you're having any problems with intercourse and whether your general health is good. Amazingly, it doesn't seem to be routine among all doctors to ask about the baby and her progress; it should be, if for no other reason than at this stage your emotional and perhaps physical health may be directly related to how she is feeding, sleeping and so on.

POST-NATAL EXERCISES Your midwife will show you these, or else a physiotherapist at the hospital will. They aren't hard or tiring, and the most difficult thing is finding the time to do them, even though they only take up five minutes a day! They are important and they can certainly help your muscles regain their tone after pregnancy and childbirth (see *pelvic floor exercises*).

POST-PARTUM HAEMORRHAGE A heavy loss of blood from the uterus after delivery. It's not common, and it can be dangerous unless it is treated promptly.

PRE-ECLAMPSIA This used to be known as toxaemia, or pre-eclamptic toxaemia. It's a condition that occurs in pregnancy and at no other time, and it disappears after the baby is born. It's not clearly understood, but it's known that around 10 per cent of first-time mothers get it, and that it's much less common in second or subsequent pregnancies. It tends to develop in the last three months or so, and the symptoms are raised blood pressure, protein in the urine and swelling round legs, ankles, face and hands (due to fluid retention). It could be linked with a calcium deficiency. If pre-eclampsia becomes more severe, it can be hazardous to the baby as there is a possibility that the placenta may cease to function properly. Severe pre-eclampsia is characterised by headaches, dizziness and sickness, and though many cases of pre-eclampsia remain mild, and harmless, they can develop into the severe sort. In true eclampsia, mother and baby risk fits and placental abruption. There is no real treatment for pre-eclampsia except rest. Occasionally drugs may be given to bring the blood pressure down. A controversial view is that it can be helped, and treated, by dietary changes, specifically by increasing the salt and protein content of your food intake. This view is not accepted by most obstetricians, who will recommend admission to hospital in many cases, and who may induce, or deliver by caesarean section the babies who seem to be at risk.

PREGNANCY Childbirth writer and antenatal teacher Sheila Kitzinger (five daughters, four pregnancies) says 'pregnancy is the only sport I've ever been any good at'. She acknowledges that some women find it a chore, but the quotation highlights the sheer 'physicalness' of being pregnant! It is *not* unusual to feel marvellously energetic, and super-healthy, at least some of the time, and to look pretty good, too.

PREPPING A midwives' term, meaning the sort of preparation you are given when you come into hospital to have your baby. There are usually standard procedures in most hospitals, and you should ask about them in advance. If you don't like the idea of any of them, then you should say so. Prepping may involve any or all of these: examination to assess how far on in labour you are; a check on the baby's heart beat; taking of your history (how long you've been in labour, whether you've noticed your waters breaking, whether there's been any bleeding etc); *bath, shave, enema,* changing into *hospital gown,* artificial rupture of *membranes* – the last four items unnecessary in many cases.

PRE-TERM BABY A baby born before 'term' – term being the full length of pregnancy. Practically speaking, it's a baby born before 37 weeks of pregnancy, and the phrase is superceding the older description 'premature'.

Pre-term babies often have special needs, and they may need admission to a *special care baby unit* or even *intensive care*. Generally, the sooner a baby's born, the more problems he's going to have, but this isn't always the case. A 33-week baby may be stronger and fitter than a 35-week baby who is also *light-for-dates*. And pre-term girls are thought to be 'tougher' than boys. Very early babies are likely to have breathing difficulties and many have feeding problems too.

There is a lot you can do for your pre-term

PRIMIGRAVIDA

baby, however, even if you feel the expert medical care he needs is taking precedence over the love and security you can give him. Research has shown that pre-term babies given contact with their mothers (stroking, nappy changing, talking, touching, feeding where possible) respond well, and make better progress than babies deprived of it. It's as if these tiny ones know they're loved and wanted, and thrive better because of it. These days many SCBUs encourage parental involvement and unrestricted visiting. The staff will help you learn how to express breast milk, and make sure your baby gets the chance to learn your feel and smell, even if he isn't strong enough to suck from the breast. The outlook for pre-term babies is better than ever it was, though a baby who was born too soon will be watched throughout his early months, and you'll be told that he's likely to reach his milestones – stages of development – slightly later than a full-term baby (see *respiratory distress syndrome*).

PRIMIGRAVIDA A woman pregnant for the first time. Some doctors still use the horrible phrase 'elderly primigravida' for anyone much over the average age having a first baby – i.e. more than 30.

PRIMIPARA A woman giving birth for the first time. During your pregnancy, your notes may describe you as para 0 if you have never given birth, para 1 if you have had one child, para 2 if you have had two children and so on.

PROGESTERONE One of the essential hormones in the life of a woman and throughout pregnancy in particular. The *corpus luteum* and then the *placenta*, after about the 14th week of pregnancy, produces it.

PROLACTIN Another hormone from the pituitary gland, mainly responsible for breast milk production after delivery.

PROLAPSE The descent of one or more of the structures of the pelvis due to weakness in the pelvic floor, or in one of the organs themselves. On prolapse of the uterus, the uterus protrudes into the lower part of the vagina. It used to be a lot more common than it is today, mainly because women used to have more children with shorter gaps between them, and received little or no after-care. In young, healthy, women, the condition is rare.

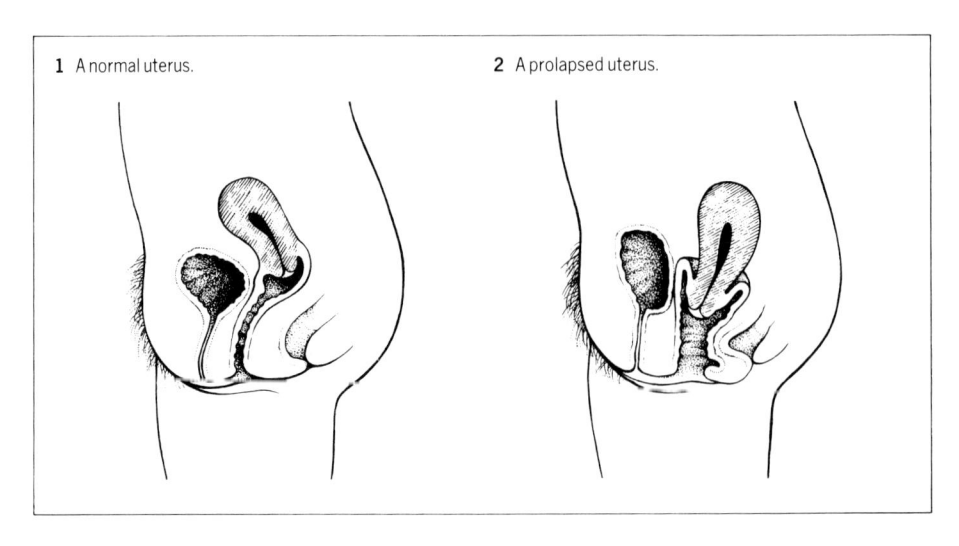

1   A normal uterus.

2   A prolapsed uterus.

PROLAPSE OF CORD This is a rare complication of labour that can happen after the waters have broken, if the head of the baby has not engaged in the pelvis. It's more common in a breech presentation. The umbilical cord has room to pass down in front of the baby's presenting part, and thereby runs the risk of being compressed as the baby descends. This is obviously life-threatening to the baby, as the cord cannot then pass oxygen to her. Once prolapse of the cord has been diagnosed the baby needs to be delivered immediately, by emergency caesarean section.

PROSTAGLANDIN A hormone used to induce labour (see *induction*).

PROTEIN IN DIET Protein-containing foods include fish, eggs, meat and animal and dairy products. Wholegrain cereals and pulses also contain protein. Protein is the 'body builder' and it's just as necessary in pregnancy as at other times. Vegetarians don't usually have a problem in getting sufficient protein as their diet includes milk, cheese, grains and pulses. Vegans avoid dairy products, so during pregnancy they need to be sure to obtain enough protein from other sources (see *diet*).

PROTEIN IN URINE The protein that's sometimes detected in the urine in pregnancy is usually albumin. Its presence can mean you have a vaginal or urine infection, or perhaps *pre-eclampsia*. Rarely, it can indicate a kidney disease.

PSYCHOPROPHYLAXIS Loosely translated, this means prevention by control by the mind. Applied to childbirth preparation, it describes a set of techniques you learn to apply during labour, to cope with the pain of contractions without drugs. These techniques may include breathing and other 'distraction' methods which, colloquially speaking, take your mind off things. Other forms of psychoprophylaxis are based on a sort of conditioned reflex where you teach your brain to interpret painful sensations as painless ones. Psychoprophylaxis has quite a respectable history and it's still widely taught, in diluted or different forms, in many countries today. The standard 'breathing and relaxation' techniques taught in UK ante-natal classes owe much to psychoprophylaxis. The drawback is however that as a method of pain relief its success varies wildly. Newer thinking on non-drugged childbirth tends to aim at total relaxation, so that mind and body are working in harmony, rather than fighting each other for the upper hand! Expectations about painless childbirth aren't raised, but women are encouraged to have the confidence in their ability to give birth joyfully and healthily. Time will tell whether this approach will give way to yet another (see *active birth; ante-natal classes; breathing in labour; natural childbirth; pain in labour; relaxation*).

PUDENDAL BLOCK A form of injected local anaesthetic which deadens the two pudendal nerves on either side of the vulva. It reduces sensation from the lower part of the vagina, the vulva, the front of the pelvic floor and the perineum. It's sometimes used when forceps are needed to deliver the baby, when the baby is already some way down the birth canal and there's no need to rotate the head.

PUERPERIUM The time after childbirth. During the puerperium you're still under the care of the *midwife* and she will check you and your baby every day, either in hospital or at home after discharge, or after a home delivery, when it will be a *community midwife* who calls, for between 10 and 28 days after your baby's birth. At some point during that time you'll be handed over to the health visitor. The midwife will look at your perineum if you have been stitched following an episiotomy, ask about and look at the *lochia*, and see how your uterus is reverting to its non-pregnant state. She'll also talk about your general health, check the baby's cord and help you with any feeding problems.

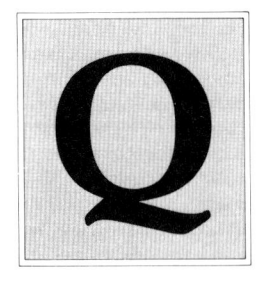

QUICKENING

QUICKENING The first sensations of movement of the unborn baby that are felt by the mother. The baby moves from very early on in pregnancy but until the movements are more vigorous, and until the uterus has some contact with the abdominal wall, you won't be able to feel them. First-time mothers don't usually recognise quickening until between the 18th and 22nd weeks; if you've had a baby before you should spot them earlier. Some mothers have described these first movements as being like a tickle on the inside; others say the movement is soft and quick, like a fish (see *fetal movements*).

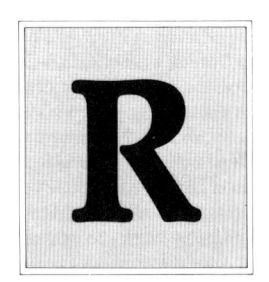

RECURRENT ABORTION This means repeated *miscarriage*, and it's also known as habitual abortion. Doctors don't usually regard miscarriage as recurrent until you've had three or more successively, but sometimes the cause of the miscarriage can be diagnosed and treatment given to prevent you miscarrying again can take place after one or two lost pregnancies. One reason for recurrent abortion could be an *incompetent cervix*.

REGISTRATION OF THE BIRTH In this country every birth must be registered, in England and Wales within 42 days of the birth, and in Scotland within 21 days. It is registered at the civic centre or town hall of the district where the baby was born. If you are married to your baby's father, either one of you can register the baby; if you are not married, you must register the birth yourself as the mother, and the baby can only be given the father's name if the father is there with you at the registration, or if you have proof of his paternity. In some big hospitals, a registrar actually comes round the maternity wards to register the births (see *birth certificate*).

RELATIONSHIPS Becoming pregnant, and then becoming a parent, doesn't just involve you in fitting another little person into your life. For most people, it leads to a sort of repositioning of yourself in relation to your parents, your grandparents, your partner and

RELATIONSHIPS

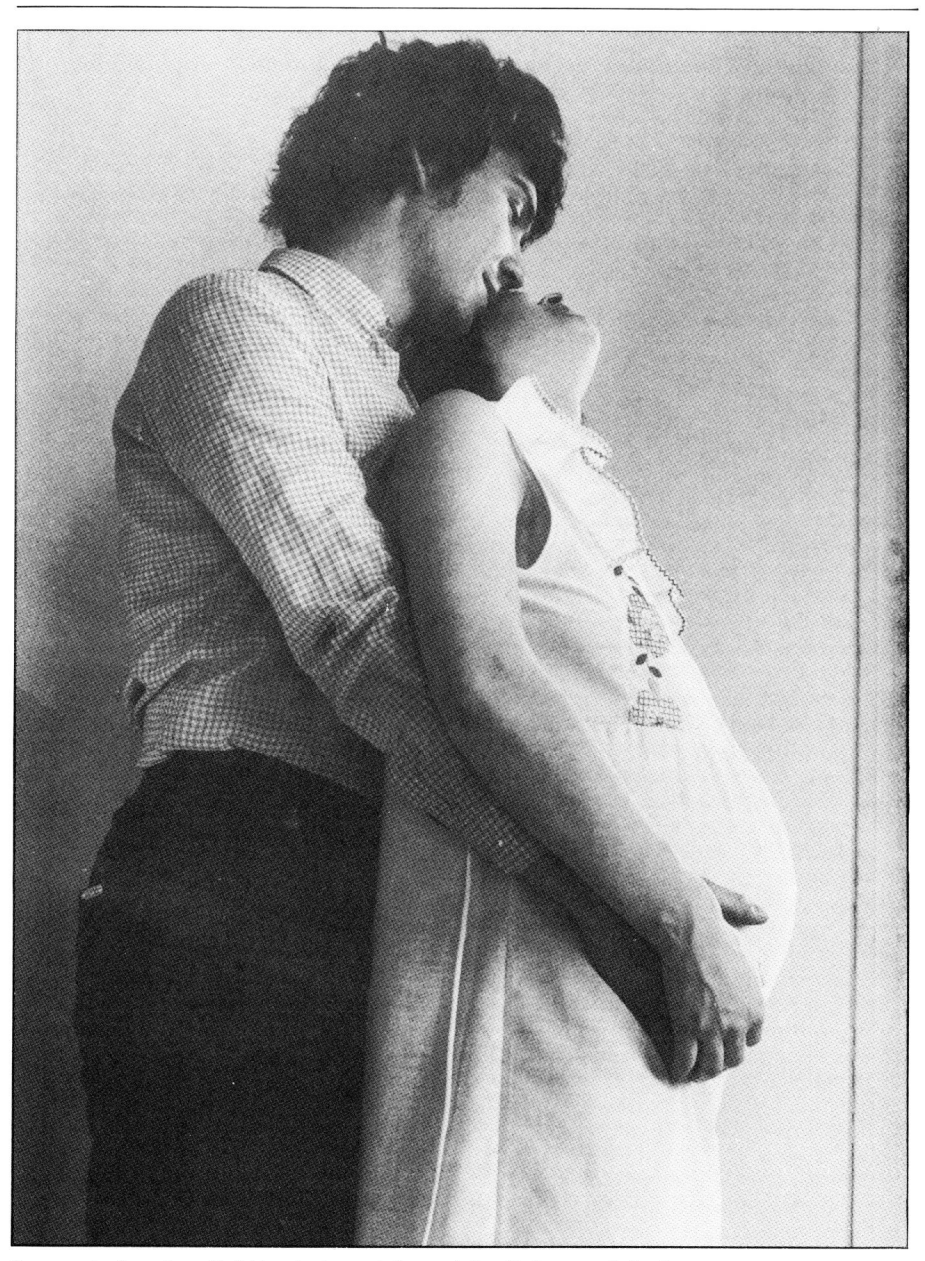

Pregnancy is often a time of heightened enjoyment of your relationship, happy and intimate.

RELAXATION

all other people you're close to. Many women, in particular, reach a better understanding with their own mothers, and become closer in many ways to other female relatives. It's as if pregnancy and birth give you an unspoken insight into the way your mother feels about you. A new baby too gives a wonderful interest that you have in common with your parents and your in-laws – maybe even the only interest you share!

The great responsibilities of a young family can so often lead to stresses and strains on a partnership that's already a bit shaky; but where a couple are committed to each other, a baby can mature and deepen the relationship they already have.

RELAXATION This is often taught as a series of simple techniques in ante-natal classes. The underlying philosophy is that pain and stress in labour are increased if a mother feels tensed up physically; on top of this, energy which could be used to actually help the baby out and to help the uterus do its job of contracting strongly and efficiently is 'used up' tensing other muscles. It's not actually a method of pain relief, more a way of helping a mother have a positive labour experience and to help her avoid feeling more tension and pain than she can cope with.

One set of techniques in common use is to consciously relax every part of your body in turn, until you are relaxed 'all over'. This state, with practice, can be reached fairly quickly when you need it. In practical terms, it means that during your labour you are not also clenching your fists, screwing up your brow and contracting your shoulder muscles at the height of a contraction; instead you are relaxed everywhere apart from your uterus (which is, of course, working involuntarily). You can practise relaxing in different positions, in preparation for moving around during labour. Relaxing slowly can be a highly effective way of getting to sleep in late pregnancy, in de-fusing any build-up of tension you feel as a reaction to hard work and stress after the baby's born, and in many other situations. It's a useful thing to learn. Many ante-natal teachers encourage relaxation techniques in combination with *breathing* methods, too (see *active birth*).

RESPIRATORY DISTRESS SYNDROME (RDS) This condition is almost never seen in full-term babies, but it's not uncommon in babies who are born several weeks too soon. It's potentially serious, and is actually the most common cause of death in *pre-term* infants. Much of the progress made in recent years in caring for tiny babies has been concerned with treating RDS, and the outlook today is getting better all the time. The major cause of RDS is immaturity of the lungs. Healthy, full-term babies produce a substance called surfactant which coats the tiny air sacs in the lungs. This means the lungs inflate and deflate easily, and breathing takes place normally, regularly and effortlessly. Pre-term babies may not produce enough surfactant, and when the air sacs deflate, the lack of surfactant makes them dry, and the walls of the air sacs stick together instead of sliding apart ready for the next breath. It's as if you had two pieces of cling film to represent two walls of an air sac. If you place a spot of detergent on each one, spread it around and then place the bits together, they won't stick to each other. A healthy baby's lungs act in the same way, with the detergent-like surfactant assisting breathing. Without detergent, the cling film sticks to the other piece, and you need more effort to pull it apart: that's what the lungs are like in a baby with RDS. Babies with RDS need to have their oxygen levels monitored and perhaps increased and they will almost certainly need help with their breathing. For this reason they are kept in *special care*. Research into the production of an artificial surfactant shows hopeful signs, but prevention of prematurity, or a reduction in it, is bound to be the most successful move against RDS.

RESPONSES OF A NEWBORN BABY The tiniest baby has certain instinctive forms of behaviour in the form of responses or reflexes

RESPONSES OF A NEWBORN BABY

that the midwife, paediatrician or obstetrician will look for. In addition to the appearance of the new baby, his general muscle tone, and the way he moves, the responses can give a good idea of his health and well-being. Some of the responses most commonly tested are the rooting reflex – when the baby's cheek is lightly touched, the baby turns his head towards the touch, seeking the nipple. If you touch his upper lip, his mouth will open and his tongue will move. Sucking is a reflex, too. The grasp reflex happens when the palm of the hand is touched (and a similar thing happens with the toes if you stroke the sole of the foot). The stepping response is shown when the baby is held in a 'standing' position. When one sole of the foot is put on a hard surface, the leg straightens out somewhat and the other foot comes forward in a stepping motion. With the Moro reflex, the baby's body and head are supported by lying across the hands and arms of the examiner, who then lets the head drop back an inch or so. The reflex action causes the baby to throw his arms out, opening his hands wide, and stretching out his legs.

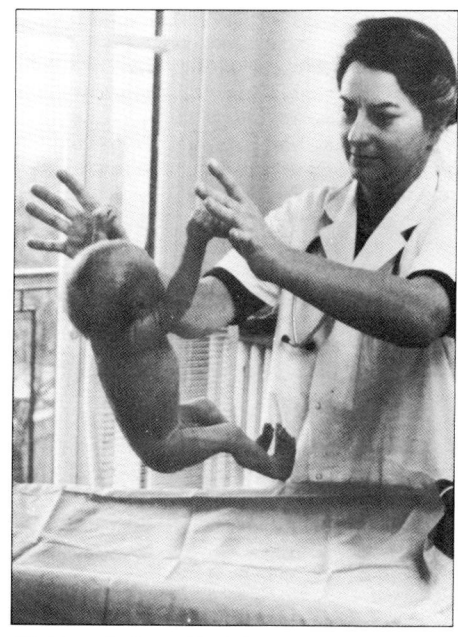

The grasp reflex is surprisingly strong.

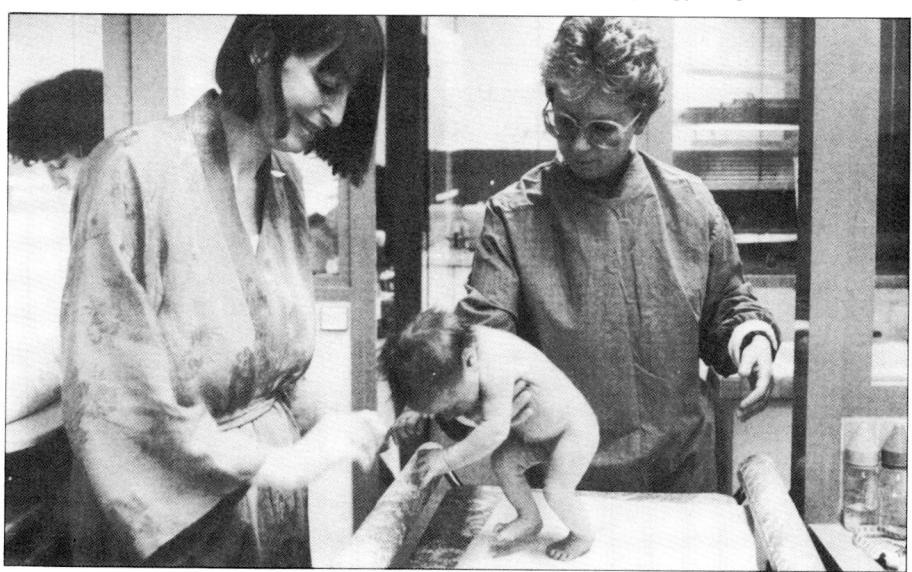

The stepping reflex is lost after a few days.

REST

REST Different books and different experts have different views about the amount of rest you should get when you're pregnant. I think for most women it's totally unrealistic to suggest (as one book does) a nine-hour sleep at night plus a two-hour nap in the day if you're having a normal pregnancy. However, if you feel you need this amount of rest, do all you can to have it. Mothers with pre-school children and working women will have to work something else out, but there's no doubt that at least some rest can make you feel better, and reduce the feeling of fatigue so many pregnant women have, particularly towards the end. Remember though that the quality, rather than the quantity, of rest is important. No use putting your feet up and then allowing anxious thoughts to get in the way of true *relaxation*. Techniques for relaxation taught at ante-natal classes can usefully be practised now, and help to make you feel satisfyingly rested (see *tiredness*).

RETAINED PLACENTA With a normal labour and birth, the placenta is expelled during the *third stage of labour*, in one or two contractions shortly after the birth of the baby. With the routine hormone injections given in this country, the third stage happens almost immediately after the birth. Occasionally, however, the placenta doesn't separate from the wall of the uterus, or it only partially separates. Or, it comes away, but isn't expelled because it is trapped within the contracted uterus, its exit closed. Prompt treatment is needed, because there is a risk of haemorrhage when the uterus isn't able to clamp down properly and shut off all its blood vessels. The treatment of retained placenta is to remove it manually, usually under general anaesthetic (see *manual removal of placenta*).

RETROVERTED UTERUS In most women, the non-pregnant uterus is anteverted – that is, it's directed towards the front of your abdomen. In a few cases, it goes the other way, and it's then described as retroverted. If you have a retroverted uterus you won't even know about it, unless a doctor carrying out an examination has told you. A pregnant retroverted uterus usually corrects itself once it rises out of the pelvic brim at the 12th week. Very occasionally this doesn't happen and the uterus becomes trapped. The main symptoms

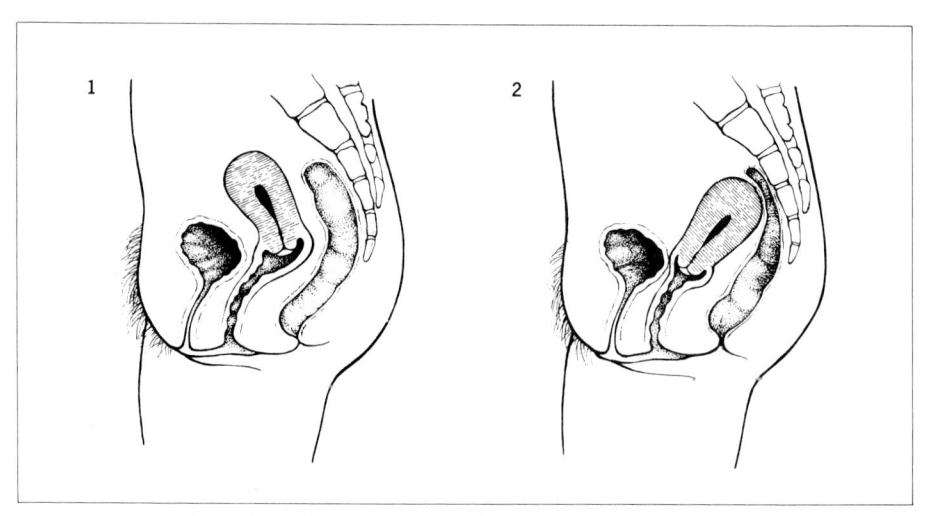

Most women have an anteverted uterus **1**. A retroverted uterus **2** is usually just a variation, and rarely causes problems.

RHESUS DISEASE

First pregnancy

Mother — Rh negative
Father — Rh positive
Baby's cells cross placenta to mother
Rh positive baby

Second pregnancy

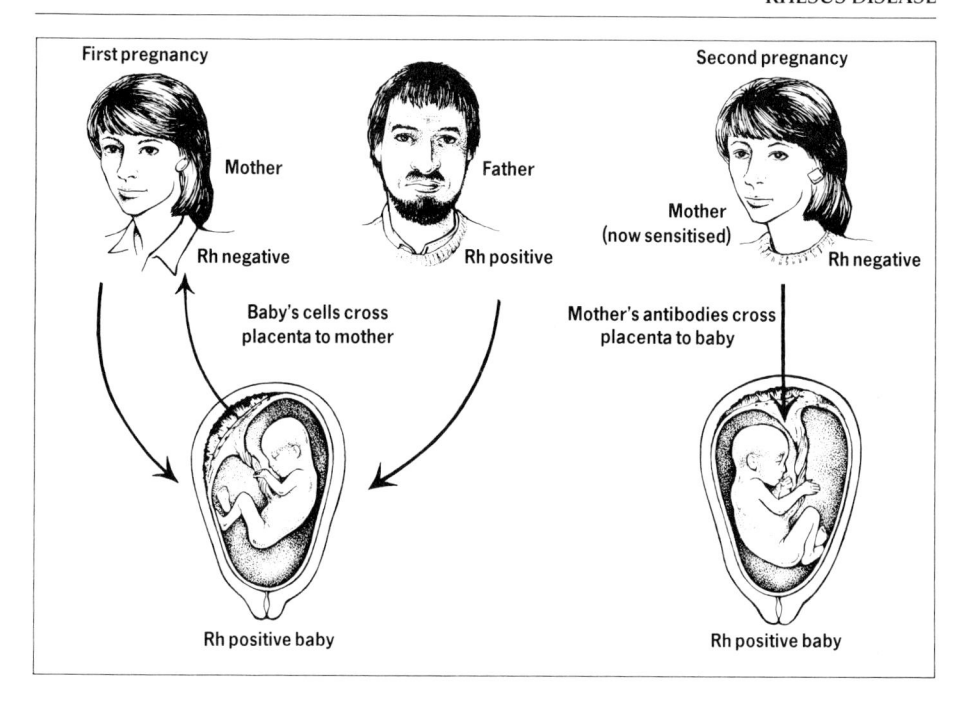

Mother (now sensitised) — Rh negative
Mother's antibodies cross placenta to baby
Rh positive baby

are pain and difficulty in passing urine. Treatment is simple: the doctor corrects the positioning of the uterus manually and may insert a plastic ring pessary to keep it in place.

RHESUS DISEASE This is also known as haemolytic disease. It's caused by Rhesus incompatability. If your red blood cells have an antigen (an immunity-producing substance) known as the Rhesus factor, your blood will be described as Rhesus positive (or Rh positive). If not, it will be described as Rhesus negative (Rh negative). Laboratory analysis of your blood will determine this one way or the other. About 85 per cent of the population are Rhesus positive; the remainder are Rhesus negative. Problems can arise when a Rhesus negative woman conceives a baby with a Rhesus positive man; the baby can therefore be either Rhesus positive or negative. During pregnancy, the mother's blood and the fetus' blood are normally completely separate, and there may be only the occasional escape of fetal blood cells into the mother's blood stream. However at delivery (or after an abortion or miscarriage), larger amounts of fetal and maternal blood cells can mix. The mother may become sensitised to the 'foreign' blood of her baby if he is Rhesus positive and develop the capacity to produce antibodies to it. If she becomes pregnant again with another Rhesus positive baby, this antibody production may get underway again and she may start, in effect, to fight against the few fetal blood cells that escape into her own circulation. These antibodies then pass to the developing fetus, and produce Rhesus disease which results in the destruction of the fetus' red blood cells. In severe cases, Rhesus disease can have serious effects, and it used to be a common cause of stillbirth or neo-natal death. The babies were known as Rhesus babies, and some were saved by a complete blood transfusion shortly after birth.

RHESUS FACTOR

Nowadays, good preventive treatment has developed, starting with discovering whether a woman is Rhesus negative or not. If she is, and her partner is too, there's no problem. If she is, and it's her first baby, there is normally no problem either (if she has had a previous abortion, stillbirth or miscarriage, however, it should be treated as her second pregnancy). She will be given an injection of a substance called Anti-D gamma globulin shortly after her baby is born, which interferes with her ability to become sensitised to the fetal blood. During her next pregnancy, her blood will be checked for antibody production (and this is sometimes done during a first pregnancy, to be on the safe side). If, for whatever reason – perhaps she didn't receive any injections – she appears to be producing antibodies, the doctor will have to gauge whether Rhesus disease is a possibility. If so, the baby may be delivered before term. Very rarely, a blood transfusion may be done while the fetus is still in the womb.

In most cases of Rhesus incompatability, the preventive measure of Anti-D injections is very successful. And when babies are born with Rhesus disease, good management means most of them can survive. There are, however, still other unsolved blood incompatabilities between a mother and her unborn baby, that preventive measures can't yet help.

RHESUS FACTOR   See *Rhesus disease.*

RIPENING OF THE CERVIX   See *cervix.*

ROOMING-IN   This is the practice of keeping mothers and babies together on the post-natal ward. The babies are usually in cribs next to the mothers' beds, and they are there all day and most nights. Sometimes, babies are taken to the nursery for the first one, two or three nights after their birth, it depends on what the policy is. If you'd prefer your baby with you all the time, however, then speak to the staff. There's no doubt that rooming-in – which is routine almost everywhere now – is far better than the separation tactics of only a few years ago, when babies were brought to their mothers at routine feeding times and that was that. With your baby right beside you you can feed whenever either of you wants to, cuddle and talk, and start getting to know each other. The main disadvantage with rooming-in is that one restless crying baby can prevent all the other mothers in the ward getting rest and sleep, unless the baby is taken to the nursery. The ideal would be for everyone to have a separate room (but then, I wonder, would you lose some of the companionship and mutual support you get from talking to the mothers near you in your ward?).

RUBELLA (GERMAN MEASLES)   When contracted in pregnancy, the rubella virus can cause great harm to an unborn baby. The baby may be born deaf, blind, with severe heart disease, mentally subnormal – and sometimes with all of these handicaps. The greatest damage is caused if the virus is caught in early pregnancy, even at times before the woman looks or feels pregnant. It can be caught by mild contact with an infected person. Women of childbearing age should make sure they are immune to rubella before they become pregnant.

In the UK a vaccination programme was started in the early 1970s, in an attempt to reach all adolescent schoolgirls. However, many were, and remain, unprotected because they didn't for some reason receive the vaccine. Women beyond their mid-20s now may not have been part of the programme anyway. This is why babies are still being born deaf, blind and profoundly handicapped because of rubella. Many more are aborted, because their mothers are discovered to have been in contact with rubella in early pregnancy.

Some women think they had rubella as a child, and are therefore immune. But rubella can be misdiagnosed, and in any case, a childhood dose does not necessarily give immunity. If you are in any doubt

SEX AFTER THE BIRTH

whatsoever, ask your doctor to arrange for a blood test to show up rubella antibodies. If the rubella antibodies are not present, or if they are in too low a concentration you'll need a vaccination at least three months before getting pregnant. The vaccine itself can damage a fetus if you don't wait this long. Because the vaccine occasionally fails, the ideal would be for every newly vaccinated woman to have a further blood test to double-check. For this to happen as routine, huge expense and organisation would be needed but GPs may be happy to arrange it on an individual basis.

Your blood is checked for rubella antibodies in early pregnancy, as part of routine blood testing. It may be shutting the stable door after the horse has bolted in that particular pregnancy, but it does mean that immediately after your baby is born, you will be given the vaccine, which will protect you in future.

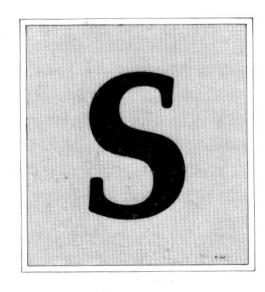

SAVAGE, Wendy In 1985 London hospital obstetrician Wendy Savage was suspended pending investigations into her 'competence'. An inquiry the following year cleared her but the case became a cause célèbre, highlighting Savage's views in favour of community-based ante-natal care, and allowing physiological labour (as opposed to high-tech intervention and caesarean section) whenever possible and whenever the mother wished it. This was contrasted with her male colleagues apparently high section rate and their opposition to 'woman-centred' obstetrics.

SCAN See *ultrasound*.

SECOND STAGE OF LABOUR The second stage of labour is when your baby is born. It starts when your cervix is fully dilated and your baby's head is ready to descend through the birth canal. You are likely to feel a strong urge to *bear down*, to help your baby on her way. Contractions continue throughout second stage, but their quality may be different from the ones you've so far experienced in first stage. They may be longer, and more close together, but because you will be aware of your body, and very aware of the fact that progress is being made, you may not experience them as painful. Standard advice to mothers in the second stage is to hold their breath and then push, as hard as possible, three enormous times during each second stage contraction. This approach is not the only one, however. A woman trying to respond to her own feelings about what her body tells her may push perhaps five or six times during a contraction, without holding her breath at all. In fact, the breath-holding that goes with exhaustive pushing can even deprive the baby of oxygen.

Positions for the second stage can vary, but an upright position of some sort allows the pelvis to open more widely, doesn't compress major blood vessels, and uses whatever help gravity can give in urging the baby downwards. The length of the second stage is normally a great deal shorter than first stage. It can occasionally be as quick as two minutes, and at the other extreme, more than two hours. Some obstetricians have a policy about 'allowing' a woman to be in the second stage only a certain amount of time before considering *forceps*. However, the most important factor should be the individual situation. If progress is being made, without signs of maternal exhaustion or fetal distress, a long second stage needn't mean intervention (see *birth position*).

SEX AFTER THE BIRTH If you haven't had stitches, if you've had a normal birth and if you feel rested and refreshed after delivery then you may want to start making love again only a few days after the birth. More

SEX IN PREGNANCY

commonly, women don't actually 'feel like it' until at least a fortnight or so afterwards, especially if they have had stitches. Some couples prefer to wait until the *lochia* has lessened. It's not at all unusual for a woman to need a few weeks or even several weeks to let her body rest, and this may especially be the case if the birth has been difficult in some way. Sex the first few times after a birth does need to be tender and slow, but most couples eventually resume a happy and loving sex life. If this doesn't happen with you, understanding and time may be all you need, so there's no need to feel anxious. If you find sex painful after childbirth tell your family doctor or health visitor. There could be a physical reason for your problem that's eminently treatable. Emotional problems with sex often solve themselves with the right conditions, but again seek help if you need it.

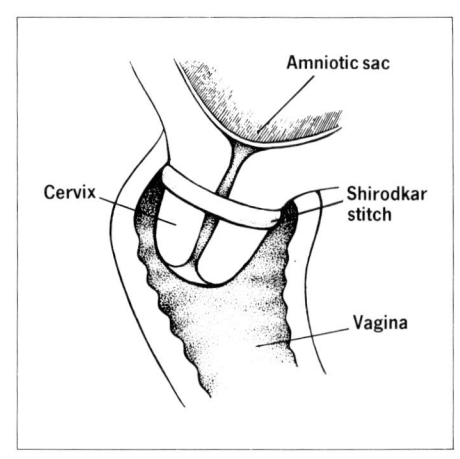

The shirodkar stitch keeps the cervix closed

SEX IN PREGNANCY See *intercourse, orgasm.*

SHARED CARE See *ante-natal care.*

SHAVE OF PUBIC HAIR In a lot of hospitals, a full or more likely partial shave of the pubic hair is a routine procedure on admittance to the labour ward. The aim is to reduce the chances of infection as the area is easier to clean when it's shaved. However, studies looking at the incidence of infections have found that shaving doesn't help at all; in fact shaving actually predisposes to infection, because of the nicks and abrasions that are inevitable. Re-growth is irritating and uncomfortable for a new mother, too. If you don't want to be shaved, tell your ante-natal clinic and have it written in your notes.

SHIRODKAR STITCH This is a drawstring type stitch that can be inserted (under anaesthetic) to keep the cervix closed where there's a possibility of *miscarriage* due to an *incompetent cervix*. It's usually put in at about the 14th week of pregnancy and taken out a week or two weeks before term.

SHOW 'Having a show' is the description of the loosening of the operculum that seals the cervix all the way through pregnancy. You may notice a pinkish blob of mucus on lavatory paper when you visit the loo, although lots of woman don't notice it because it just gets flushed away unless they've been specially looking. Having a show is a sign that labour won't be long in starting – maybe, a couple of days or so, and often much sooner (see *operculum*).

SIBLINGS Brothers and sisters. The theory is that siblings are always supposed to be jealous of each other in childhood, although this is not always the case. However, if you're pregnant with your second or subsequent child, you'll obviously need to be sensitive to your elder child's needs and accept there may be signs of upset at the prospect, and the actuality, of a new baby. In practical terms, this might mean not leaving them alone in the same room for even a second, at least until you really trust the older one not to hurt the baby. Many hospitals these days welcome visits by siblings and this is a good chance to make the first introductions. It's possible that we tend to make too much of the jealousy angle. In many cases, the love and companionship that can exist between brothers and sisters is one of the joys of family life.

SICKLE CELL DISEASE A serious form of anaemia found in people of African, Asian, Arab and West Indian descent. It's hereditary, although parents may only have the sickle cell trait, which isn't in itself harmful. If a pregnant woman has sickle cell disease her pregnancy will be watched very carefully, as pregnancy can lead to a crisis of the disease.

SICKNESS Often an early symptom of pregnancy. Fortunately for most women, it is one that disappears in the first 12 weeks. While it lasts though it can be misery-making and highly inconvenient. For some women it is just a sensation of nausea; for others it involves actual vomiting. It is frequently referred to as morning sickness, though this is misleading as it can occur at any time of the day or night. Some women find it lasts the whole way through pregnancy, and quite puts them off the idea of having another baby.

Simple measures can sometimes help. Keep your meals small and frequent, and regularly spaced throughout the day. A dry cracker and a cup of tea *before* you get out of bed (loving partner needed here) is known to help, and recent research suggests that cutting down your intake of fat, and increasing your intake of unrefined carbohydrate (wholegrains, fresh potato) taking more rest and avoiding stress can all help. Sipping sweet drinks (not fizzy ones) has helped some women too. There are

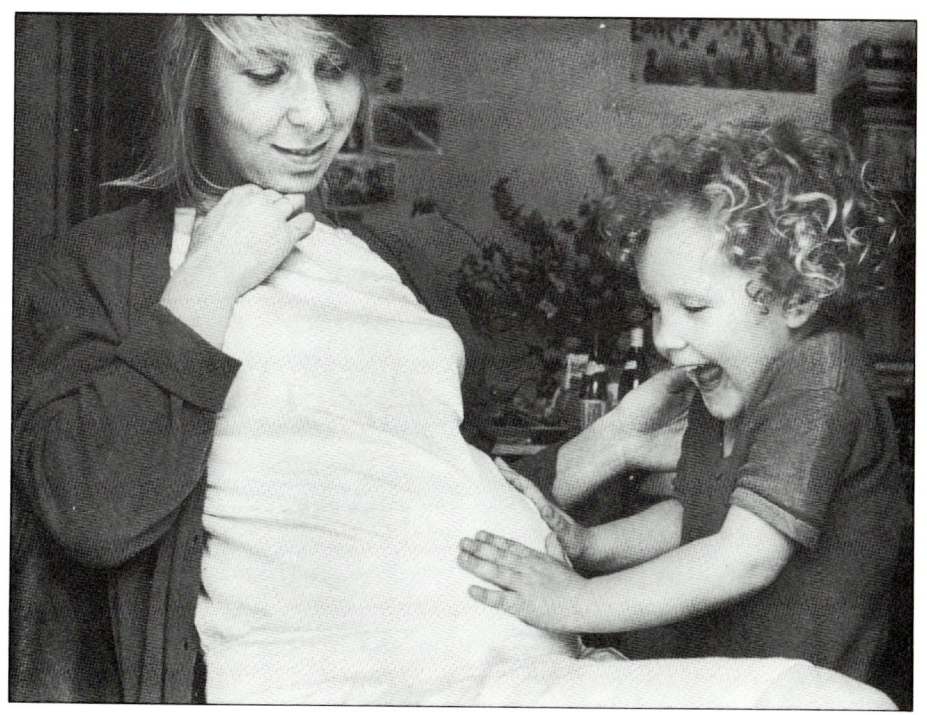

Pregnancy can be an exciting time for everyone.

SIGNS OF LABOUR

drugs available for pregnancy sickness but many doctors are understandably reluctant to prescribe them after recent scares, which linked one widely prescribed drug to birth defects here and in America.

SIGNS OF LABOUR All normal labours eventually have the strong, regular contractions that precede delivery, but few actually start off like this. The first signs of labour are more likely to be short, spaced out, irregular contractions that get gradually longer and more frequent. You may or may not notice a *show* and your waters may or may not break spontaneously before you have noticed any contractions. You may have a few hours of 'am I or aren't I?' contractions before you're sure, and false alarms aren't anything to be embarrassed about, even if you end up in hospital with them. Other possible signs to look out for are: a drop in weight a few days before labour is due; a sudden surge of energy a couple of days before labour starts; diarrhoea a few hours before labour gets underway.

SIGNS OF PREGNANCY The first and most obvious sign of pregnancy is, of course, a missed period. Other early signs are a tingling tender feeling in the *breasts*, a need to urinate more frequently, the appearance of *Montgomery's tubercles* on the nipple, possible *sickness* and *tiredness*. On an internal examination, a doctor or midwife can detect a pregnant uterus from about seven weeks.

SKIN IN PREGNANCY Your skin can look very good in pregnancy, even if you normally have the tendency to the odd spot or two. However, some women find their skin is also very itchy and dry; smoothing in a bland cream can help, as can bath oil.

SLEEP AFTER THE BIRTH You might find you're feeling too 'high' after the birth of your baby to want to sleep, and if your baby is separated from you for any reason you may feel too anxious. Eventually, though, you will want to sleep, and it's unfortunate that the post-natal ward is just about the worst place for getting any real undisturbed rest. Sleeping pills are often given at night in hospitals, and if lack of sleep is making you slow to recover, then this sort of help may be what you need. But remember that the dopey feeling you get with pills can linger on, and if you are wanting to breastfeed, you need to give night feeds anyway. There is bound to be a trace of sleeping drugs getting through to your breast milk, too. Early discharge may be the answer if you reckon you have a better chance of sleep at home.

SLEEP IN PREGNANCY See *insomnia*.

SMALL-FOR-DATES See *light-for-dates*.

SMEAR TEST A test to check for abnormal, possibly pre-cancerous cells on the cervix. The smear test is a simple and effective preventive measure against cancer of the cervix, and it's often done routinely after childbirth, or at the *post-natal examination*, or perhaps ante-natally in the clinic. A small scraping is quite painlessly taken from the surface of your cervix during an *internal examination* and then sent on a small glass slide to the laboratory.

SMOKING Smoking in pregnancy is associated with low-birthweight in the baby, plus an increased risk of stillbirth and neo-natal death. This seems to be because nicotine prevents the placenta working at full efficiency, which reduces its ability to help a fetus to remain healthy and to grow well. Smoking also reduces your general health by robbing your body of vitamins and minerals – and your own state of health and nutrition has an effect on the health of your baby. However, smoking can be a difficult habit to break and you may need help. Remember it's never too late to stop as the effects of smoking are worse

SPECIAL CARE

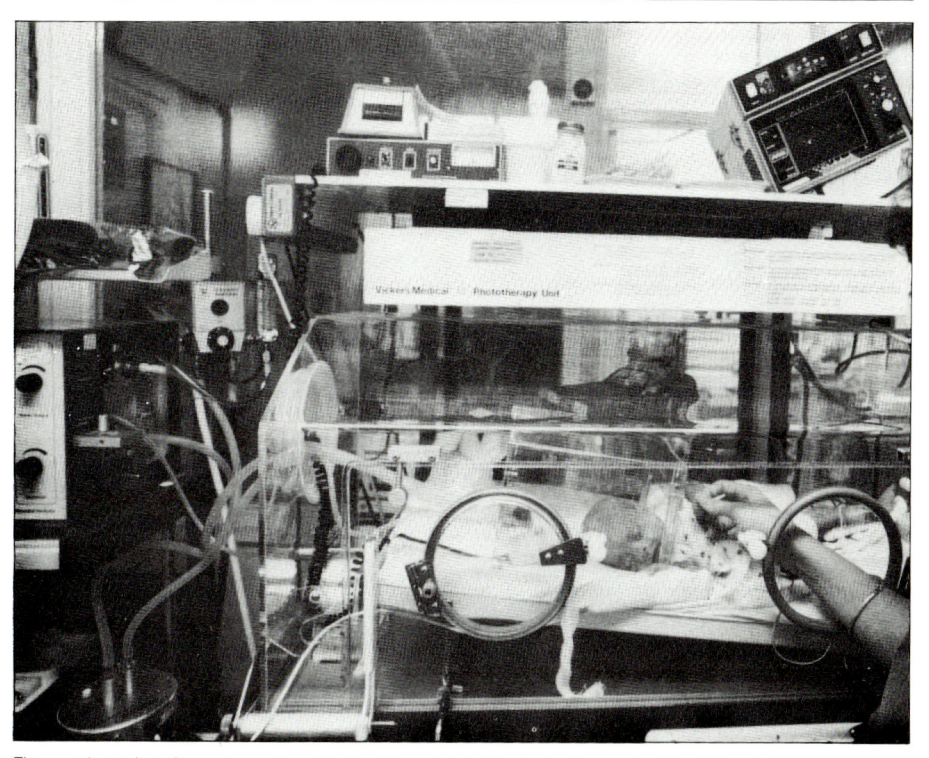

The complicated machinery may seem like a barrier, but even tiny, sick babies need your touch and love.

towards the end of pregnancy. Take comfort from the fact that cutting down – if you really can't give up – does make a difference, and if you can get down to under ten a day, the worst effects of smoking will be minimised.

SORE NIPPLES A miserable complication of breastfeeding. Making sure your baby's *latching on* correctly is the important preventive factor. If you do get sore, a midwife or breastfeeding counsellor can check the baby's position and give advice on healing. Keeping nipples dry between feeds helps.

SPECIAL CARE Hospitals delivering babies almost always have Special Care Baby Units (SCBUs) where tiny, sick or pre-term infants can be looked after especially vigilantly. Latest figures show that around one in seven newborns spends some time in special care, but this includes babies brought in for an hour or so simply for observation, plus babies with *jaundice,* who are otherwise well, but who need 'the lights'. There are some murmurings that babies are taken into the SCBU unnecessarily when both mother and baby would be better off staying together. Whether this is the case or not, there's no doubt that many babies do benefit greatly from the close attention and nursing and medical care in the SCBU, and parents themselves are much more likely to be welcomed as a vital part of this care than they used to be. It's easy to feel anxious and even stunned when your baby needs special care, particularly if she needs help with her breathing and feeding, and needs constant monitoring. Talk to the nurses and doctors; ask how long your baby will need special care and get them to explain all the tests and machines to you.

SPHYGMOMANOMETER The device used to measure your *blood pressure* (known as a 'sphygmo').

SPINA BIFIDA One of the neural tube defects. Spina bifida babies have a major defect of the spine, and in the most severe cases part of the spinal cord is exposed, without any covering of skin or bone. In milder cases there may simply be some bone missing in one of the vertebrae of the spinal column. Children born with severe spina bifida are paralysed and they may be mentally handicapped as well. An operation to close the open part of the cord will decrease the likelihood of the baby dying from infection, but even so, spina bifida can be fatal.

In some cases, though, the outlook isn't so gloomy. Many children will need constant care, and possibly a series of operations, but the degree of handicap is very variable and not always predictable. Once you have had one child with spina bifida, you are statistically more likely to have another with either this or another neural tube defect. *Genetic counselling* will help you assess the risks.

SPOTTING Very light bleeding – showing up as small spots of blood on your pants – that sometimes happens in pregnancy. It can precede heavier bleeding which is potentially serious, but in many cases the spotting ceases and the pregnancy continues perfectly normally. You should seek medical advice, however, if it happens.

SQUATTING See *birth positions*.

STICKY EYE This is a very common irritation or infection in the first few days of a baby's life. Either one or both eyes are affected by a discharge of pus that can 'glue' the upper and lower eyelids together. It's usually not known for certain how the condition has been picked up but it's rarely anything serious. In hospital the paediatrician may decide to take swabs for the laboratory to check over, and you may be given a special antibiotic ointment or drops to apply to your baby's eyes. Often, however, careful wiping of your baby's eyes with a weak salt solution (provided by the hospital) clears it up very quickly.

STILLBIRTH The delivery of a baby who has already died in the uterus after 28 weeks of pregnancy (sooner than this, and it's termed a late miscarriage). The causes of stillbirth are various: they include abnormalities in the baby, early separation of the placenta (so the placenta comes away before the baby is born), *placental insufficiency* and certain infections that the mother has had which have crossed the placental barrier. In some cases, no obvious cause is found. Parents of a stillborn child need to grieve, and the experience of parents who have come through this tragedy suggests most strongly that they have a need to see and hold their dead baby. A photograph can help them to mourn, and to have some tangible reminder of the child they have loved even though they have not had the chance to 'know' their baby like other parents. Parents can arrange for a funeral, but even if they don't, it can be a comfort to know exactly where their baby is buried, and parents should let the hospital know they wish to have this knowledge, if it's the hospital making the arrangements. You can get support and love from friends and family – or from other parents of stillborn children (see Useful Addresses).

STITCHES If you have an *episiotomy*, which is a cut made in the perineum, when your baby is born, or if you tear more than just slightly, you will need stitches (also called sutures) to join the tissues up again. If you have had a local anaesthetic injection when the episiotomy was made and you don't have to wait too long to be stitched, stitching shouldn't hurt at all. If it does, tell the doctor. It's a simple matter to give you another dose of anaesthetic, and there's absolutely no reason, after all, why you should be allowed to feel the tiniest pinprick. The doctor, rather than the midwife, is likely to stitch you up if you are in hospital. Many of the problems associated with episiotomy are in fact as a result of the way a mother has been stitched up, and doctors are under a real obligation to take extra special care. If the episiotomy or tear is a deep or extensive one, it can take up to an hour to stitch, but the 'average' cut probably only needs half an hour or so. These days suturing material is almost invariably designed to dissolve harmlessly after healing has taken place, so there is no need to have the stitches removed. Some women find their stitches very uncomfortable in the days following the birth; it's often described as 'sitting on thorns'. Sitting on a child's blow-up swimming ring can help. Also ask the midwife to take a look at the stitches (which she will do on a daily basis anyway) in case there's a particularly spiky one she can trim for you. Sometimes a mild painkiller, like paracetemol, can help; your hospital will have supplies. A mild salt solution douche (squirted from a squeezy bottle) promotes healing of the perineum. Keep the area dry – drying off with a hair dryer after a bath is gentler than a towel.

STRESS INCONTINENCE Sometimes a cough or a sneeze or running upstairs, or a fit of laughing, can cause your bladder to leak a small amount. It seems, too, that this isn't a rare problem among pregnant or newly-delivered women. The cause is usually a weakness of the pelvic floor muscles; when these muscles are relaxed suddenly, the consequent loss of tone allows the urine to escape. The problem often cures itself a few weeks after delivery, but it can be very much helped by *pelvic floor exercises* to increase the muscle tone. If time and exercise don't help, see your doctor.

STRETCH MARKS You may get them – you may not. It doesn't seem to make any difference whether you lard yourself with anti-stretch mark cream through pregnancy or not. Some women who get absolutely mountainous in pregnancy seem to escape them, while others with only the tiniest bump at nine months get landed with dozens. Stretch marks is a pretty accurate description, as they are the result of the elastic-like fibres in the lower layers of the skin stretching and breaking beyond repair. They start off as pink or pinkish-blue lines on your tummy (and sometimes breasts) and as time goes on they fade to a silvery-white colour and become much less noticeable. Why some women get them and others don't is a mystery. It could be something to do with the sort of skin type you were born with, or it could be that a good healthy diet may do more than anything else to prevent them.

SUGAR IN URINE One of the substances your urine is tested for during pregnancy is sugar. Its presence is often insignificant, but it can sometimes indicate *diabetes*.

SUITCASE FOR HOSPITAL If you're planning a hospital delivery, your ante-natal clinic may give you a list of the things they expect you to bring in. If not, then it's helpful to think in two categories: what you need for labour and birth, and then what you'll need afterwards, which will partly depend on the length of your stay. Don't forget that if you're expecting daily visitors during your stay, they can bring in things like clean nighties and towels as you need them. On the day you go home, your visitor can bring in your outdoor clothes as well.

Here's a checklist to remind you of what you'll need:
For labour (keep separate in a small bag or

119

SWELLING

case from the rest of your gear) – two nighties; slippers; two flannels (for the nurse or midwife to wash you afterwards); comb and slides to tie long hair out the way; small natural sponge for moistening face and lips; flask of honeyed or glucose water; food for partner; toilet bag; pants; towel.
For afterwards – nighties; lightweight dressing gown or bedjacket; sanitary towels (unless hospital provides them); cosmetics; reading matter; letter paper; coins for pay phone; pants (choose disposable paper pants, or old pants you won't mind throwing away).

SVD Seen on notes, it simply means spontaneous vaginal delivery – a normal delivery without forceps or induction or section.

SWELLING See *oedema*.

SYNTOCINON The brand name of synthetic *oxytocin*, given (usually) as a drip. It stimulates the uterus to contract and therefore starts off labour or hastens its progress.

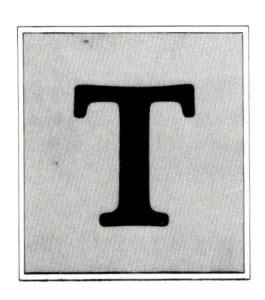

TEAR IN PERINEUM The perineum can become so thinned out during delivery of the baby that it tears. General opinion is still that an *episiotomy* can prevent a tear, or that it's better to have a straight episiotomy than a jagged tear, but recent studies throw doubt on this, in terms of the length of time needed for the wound to heal. It's not uncommon to have an episiotomy and a tear, and small tears appear to heal better than episiotomies on the whole. Skilled midwifery – mainly the careful management of the delivery of the head and shoulders – lessens the chance of a bad tear. All but the smallest tears need stitching.

TEETH IN PREGNANCY In the UK, you are entitled to free dental treatment during pregnancy and for a year after your baby is born. Tell your dentist if you are having treatment when you think you might be pregnant, so he can avoid giving you X-rays. A good diet and a thorough cleaning routine are even more important for maintaining healthy teeth and gums during pregnancy.

TERM A baby born at 'term' is born when he or she is expected. Strictly speaking, term is the exact expected day, and if your baby is born a few (say three) days before or after, you may have 'T−3' or 'T+3' on your notes. More generally, however, a term baby is born at somewhere around the 40 week mark (within a fortnight or so either side) and on this basis most babies are in fact born at term.

THALASSAEMIA An inherited form of anaemia, mainly found in people from Mediterranean countries and parts of Asia.

THIRD STAGE OF LABOUR This is normally thought of as the final stage of labour, during which the placenta and membranes are delivered, with one or two contractions. In this country, the third stage happens a few minutes after delivery, because most women are given a routine injection of a drug called syntometrine, which causes the uterus to contract and expel the remaining contents. Left to themselves, most women's third stage would perhaps happen 10 or 20 minutes later (sometimes longer). The uterus contracts by itself, under the stimulus of the baby's sucking at the breast which produces natural oxytocin. Because syntometrine works so quickly and effectively, the placenta needs to be out before the lower part of the uterus contracts so strongly that the placenta gets trapped inside. Midwives usually make sure this happens by means of 'controlled cord traction' whereby the cord is drawn out, bringing the placenta with it. This sort of active management of the third stage is aimed at reducing the risks of *post-partum haemorrhage*. The syntometrine also closes off the blood vessels inside the uterus, which prevents excessive bleeding.

However the process isn't without risks of its own. There is a risk of a trapped placenta (which has to be removed under general anaesthetic): of traction leaving behind a piece of afterbirth; or a badly executed traction actually turning the uterus inside out. There is room for differences of opinion about the net benefits in routine active management of the third stage. Complications can occur when it is actively managed – and when it isn't. In virtually all hospitals in the West, however, active management is absolutely routine (see *cutting the cord*).

THREATENED MISCARRIAGE A possible but not definite miscarriage. Bleeding from the vagina in pregnancy is always potentially serious, but if the bleeding stops, and the cervix has remained closed, the miscarriage has been a 'threatened' one rather than actual.

THROMBOSIS A thrombosis is a clot of blood in a vein. It may occur in the legs when it happens in pregnancy or soon after childbirth. Superficial thrombosis is the more common type, and it's unlikely to cause any problem apart from an aching pain in the affected area of the leg. It starts with a *varicose vein* in most cases, and the treatment is exercise of the leg, plus support with a firm bandage or support stocking.

Deep vein thrombosis happens more rarely, affecting a deep vein of the leg. It's potentially more serious and treatment is likely to involve a support bandage and an anti-coagulant drug to prevent the clot dislodging and ending up in a lung (causing pulmonary embolism). One of the reasons why you'll be encouraged to get up a few hours after the birth of your baby is to avoid thrombosis. If you're not allowed up (perhaps after a caesarean section) straight away, you'll be shown how to do ankle exercises.

THRUSH A vaginal infection, causing a white discharge, which is quite common in pregnancy, particularly if you've had it before. It causes annoying itching. The doctor can prescribe pessaries which clear it up in a few days (your partner should be treated too, in recurrent attacks). A natural remedy is to insert live yoghurt (from health shops); it's messy but effective. Help to prevent further bouts by avoiding nylon tights and pants. Other names for thrush are monilia and candida.

TIREDNESS A certain amount of tiredness is normal in early pregnancy particularly, and then later on towards the end. An increased feeling of fatigue may well be your body 'telling' you to slow down and have a rest. It could also be a sign that your diet could be improved. This goes for later pregnancy too, and the feeling of tiredness is exacerbated by the fact that you're having to lug an extra weight around with you all the time. Having said that, there are women who seem to be very energetic all the way through pregnancy.

It's important – for both you and your growing baby – to rest when you feel you need to. This isn't always easy, and you may need to involve friends or relatives in looking after older children, or to seek other help so you don't always spend your lunch hour at work tearing round the shops. Tell your ante-natal clinic or doctor if you feel constantly tired.

TNS (or TENS) This stands for 'transcutaneous nerve stimulation'. It's a method of pain-relief that has been used in cases of non-childbirth related pain for some time. It works by transmitting electrical

TOPPING AND TAILING

impulses from a small battery-operated plastic box attached to electrodes that are taped to the patient's skin. In childbirth, it's recently been tried out as an alternative to other forms of pain-relief, and as it's administered by the mother herself and doesn't interfere with her ability to change position or walk around, and doesn't appear to have a negative effect on the baby, it may turn out to have a future. It's not at all clear why a series of self-imposed electrical shocks (however mild) should reduce awareness of pain; it could be something to do with the distracting effect, or perhaps the impulse stimulates the body to release its own natural pain-relievers.

TOPPING AND TAILING This is something you'll be shown by a midwife. It's a way of keeping your baby's face, ears, neck, hands and nappy area clean without actually bathing her. It's quite simple, requiring cotton wool and a bowl of warm water. You top her first, by taking dampened cotton wool swabs over her face, round her neck and ears, and eyes (if *'sticky'*, use clean, separate pieces of cotton wool for each eye – and wipe from the inside of the eye outwards). Then do her hands and underarms. Tailing is washing the bottom (make sure you reach the folds round her thighs). You should always make sure your baby's skin is dried gently and thoroughly, as a new baby's skin is prone to rashes and soreness.

TOXAEMIA See *pre-eclampsia*.

TRANQUILLISERS These are not advisable in pregnancy, if they can possibly be avoided. The main problem is that they can actually cause withdrawal symptoms in a new baby, as well as convulsions and feeding problems. Tranquillisers are sometimes given to help a woman in early labour who is frightened and agitated. In extreme cases, this sort of one-off dose could therefore be justified.

TRANSITION A term sometimes used to describe a period between first stage and second stage of labour – between the full dilatation of the cervix and the urge to bear down. Not all women experience it. For those that do it usually lasts a few minutes (although it can be shorter or longer) and you may find it the hardest part of your labour (not helped by the practice in many hospitals of using this moment to put you on a trolley bound for the delivery room), and you may become irritable and angry with the medical staff and your partner. Some women report that their emotions are confused and a calm, loving and supportive partner is invaluable. Other women speak of total relaxation at this stage, while they wait to welcome the powerful bearing down sensations that are bound to come. The contractions during transition may be felt as the longest ones of your labour, and they come very frequently. You aren't able to bear down with them, so you will need to aim much more consciously at being relaxed and comfortable.

TRANSVERSE LIE A baby in the uterus can lie across it instead of upwards or downwards. Unless he changes position before labour, he will present by the shoulder which means a caesarean section will have to be carried out. Occasionally the second born of twins manages to get himself into this position when waiting to be born.

TRIAL OF LABOUR Obstetricians may decide on a trial of labour when it's not clear whether a mother will be able to deliver vaginally or not. This may happen when there's some doubt as to the size and shape of the pelvis or some sort of difficult situation during delivery with a previous baby. You may be told that going into labour normally is fine, but that you will be watched and the progress of your labour and the health of your baby monitored, in case it seems a caesarean section will be needed after all. If you have had a previous caesarean section, for a reason that's not expected to happen again, a vaginal

TWINS

delivery may well be possible and this is more properly termed a 'trial of scar'.

Try and get the chance to discuss trial of labour or scar with your doctor, to find out what he would expect to happen or not to happen, before he considered a caesarean section to be the inevitable course. If you're happy for him to say, 'Well, we'll see how you get on,' then that's fair enough. But if you want to be really clear, you'll need to know whether he's going to be concentrating on timing the labour rather than assessing its progress. The trouble with 'trials' of this sort is that a woman can feel exactly as if she's on trial herself! Instead of having a normal labour, she may end up watching the clock anxiously, and being worried about whether her contractions are strong and frequent enough to satisfy the doctor. This sort of anxiety in itself can interfere with the progress of labour. Even so it should be encouraging to note that given the chance many women with previous caesareans can deliver vaginally next time round.

TRILENE A form of pain-relief in labour given through a mask over your face. You use it like *Entonox* – and, in fact, because Entonox has none of the disadvantages of trilene (which has a build-up effect), trilene is used less and less today.

TRIMESTER For convenience, the approximate nine months of pregnancy are divided up into three trimesters of three months each – the first, second and third trimesters respectively.

TRIPLETS Triplets occur in every 9000 births. Like *twins*, they can be identical or from three separate acts of fertilisation. Sometimes, they can be formed of a set of identical twins and one singleton. Much of the information given in the entry for twins applies to triplets, including the fact that it's perfectly possible with the right help and support, to breastfeed triplets, though some mothers of triplets find a combination of bottles and breasts easier to cope with.

TROPHOBLAST The trophoblast is developed from the fertilised egg, and it eventually forms the placenta and membranes. It starts to develop only a few days after conception, and it is responsible for the pregnancy embedding in the lining of the uterus.

It may be that the trophoblast will become important in ante-natal testing for some abnormalities. It's been known for some time that the trophoblast starts shedding some of its cells in the second week after fertilisation. These cells mingle with the mother's bloodstream. Researchers have developed a special antibody that sticks to trophoblast cells, and no others in the mother's blood. This means that if a small sample of blood is taken from the mother (just as in any other routine blood test) it can have its trophoblast cells hived off. These cells can then be studied for genetic abnormalities – as, of course, the trophoblast has exactly the same genetic formation as the fetus. It's expected that the sort of information obtained will be the same as the information currently available from *amniocentesis* and *chorion biopsy*. But there are great, potential advantages over either of these two tests: a sampling of the mother's blood is far simpler and less invasive than amniocentesis or chorion biopsy; there is no risk at all of harming mother or baby; and if, as a result, genetic abnormalities are shown, discussion can take place and abortion offered at a far earlier stage. The test is still in its very early experimental phases, and it's unlikely to be generally available for some time. However, as a technique for the future it shows promise.

TWINS Twins happen approximately every 80 pregnancies. If you, the mother, have twins in your family, especially on your mother's side, then your chances are increased. Twins are of two types: monozygotic or uniovular, which are identical, or dizygotic or binovular,

123

TWINS

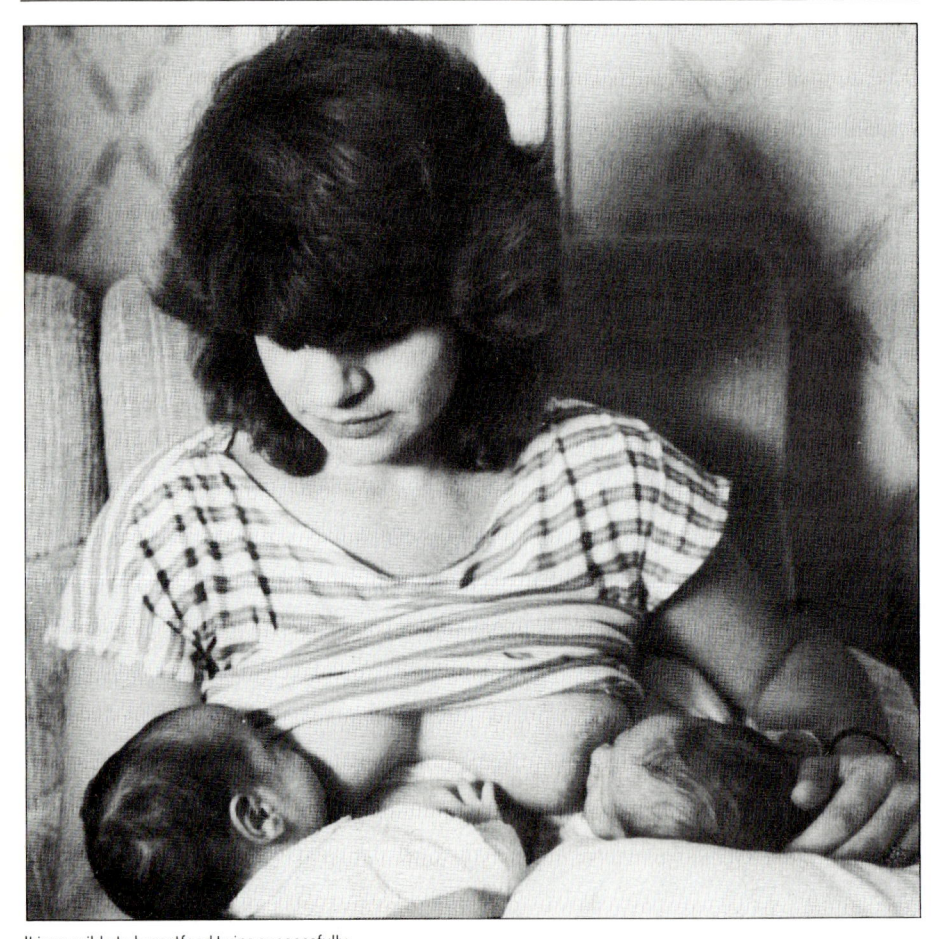

It is possible to breastfeed twins successfully.

which are no more alike than you'd expect brothers and sisters to be anyway. Identical twins are always of the same sex, and they have developed from one egg and fertilised by one sperm which splits into two. Non-identical twins are the inherited sort, and they are three times more common than identical twins. They develop as a result of two eggs being fertilised by two sperm.

Most twins these days are diagnosed before delivery. Generally, the ante-natal clinic will notice an unusual weight gain, and a larger-than-usual uterus. Later on, the midwife may hear two quite separate heart beats. When there's any suspicions, you'll be asked to go for an ultrasound scan which will resolve the issue.

A twin delivery has increased risks for mother and babies, and a hospital confinement is normally the best option. One of the risks is prematurity; another is malpresentation (where at least one of the

124

ULTRASOUND

twins is in a less-than-ideal position). Sometimes, one twin may be a lot smaller than the other and need special attention at birth and after. Labour isn't necessarily longer with twins than with a single baby, except where there are complications due to malpresentation.

Twins are obviously harder work to look after in the early days, but don't let anyone tell you you won't be able to breastfeed, if this is what you want to do. More and more mothers of twins are breastfeeding very successfully, and finding it more convenient than bottle feeding would be. With the right sort of encouragement and practical help, breastfeeding works very well (see Useful Addresses).

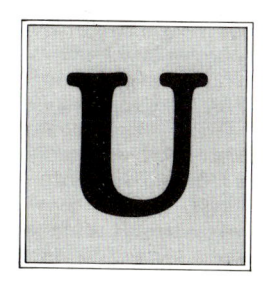

U

ULTRASOUND Ultrasound scanning has quickly become a part of routine ante-natal care in most large hospitals, over a surprisingly short period of ten or fifteen years. It's highly sophisticated technology, and it enables the contents of your uterus to be

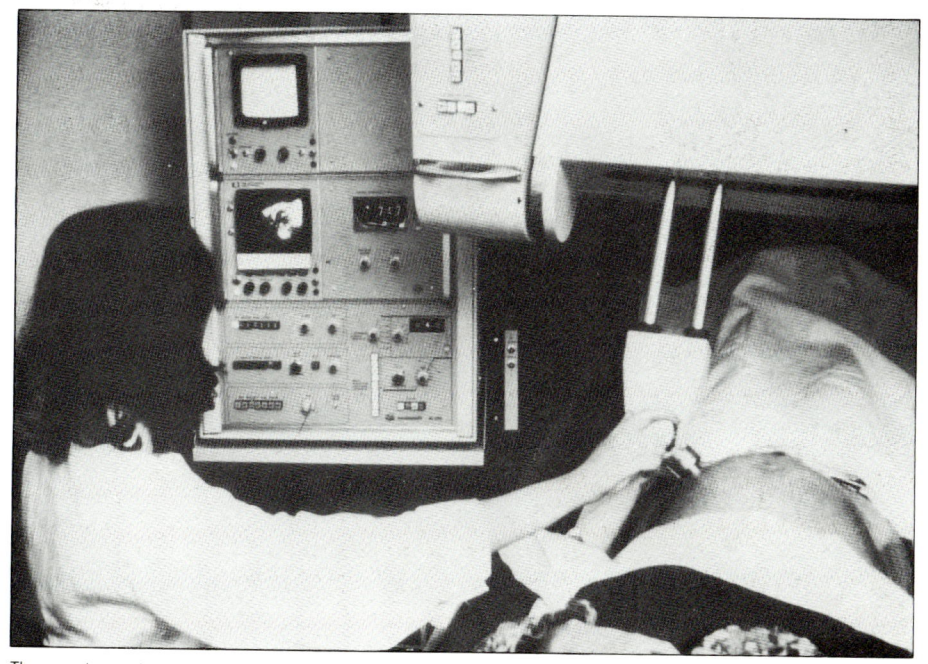

The scanning equipment produces a 'picture' on the screen.

125

ULTRASOUND

looked at without X-ray. The basis of ultrasound relies on soundwaves. Each surface of the object being looked at by ultrasound will reflect different soundwaves, and this is transferred to a screen in graphic form. Both the upper and lower surface of the object will be represented, so if you were looking at a hot dog with ultrasound you'd see the upper surface of the top layer of the bread; lower surface of the top layer of the bread; top surface of sausage; bottom surface of the sausage; upper surface of the bottom layer of the bread; lower surface of the bottom layer of the bread. Looking at a fetus and placenta is enormously more complicated, and you need to be especially trained to interpret the scan of a pregnant uterus. That's why, even when the doctor or radiographer takes the trouble to point out to you various bits of your baby on the screen, you may still see a black, white and grey series of splodges. By measuring the fetus, comparing the scan to any previous ones and looking at the formation of the spine and other organs, the growth and development of the fetus can be checked. You can also check for twins (or more). Ultrasound also pinpoints the position of the placenta (to diagnose *placenta praevia* and to ascertain the right place for the syringe in *amniocentesis*).

There is a 'but' to all this technological marvel, though. While almost everyone agrees that ultrasound can be a useful, even vital, diagnostic tool, doubts are being expressed about its growing routine use. In some units, all pregnant women are scanned at least once, and some are scanned many times. Laboratory work in America, however, suggests that ultrasound waves could cause long-term damage to cells, and this work has caused some American experts to be very wary of ultrasound. In this country, doctors are more cautious about accepting the validity of this

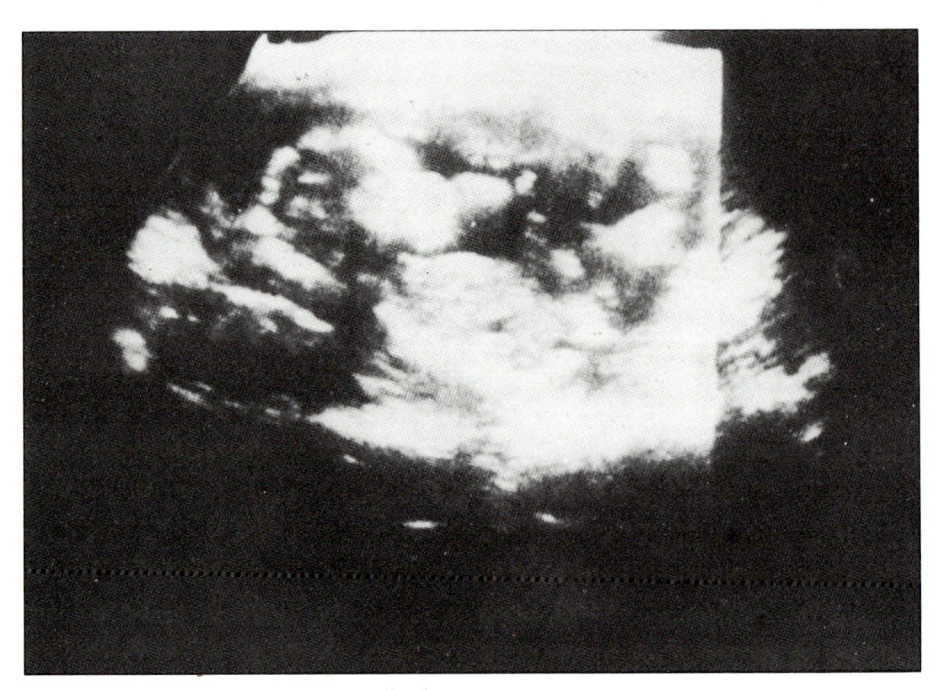

The fetus, 18 weeks old, is clearly seen sucking its thumb.

research and of its relevance to humans in real-life conditions. They point out the machines used in obstetrics send out only short pulses of ultrasound; the machines are designed to avoid the possibility of larger 'doses'. However, many doctors have not been at all cautious in pressing ahead with routine use of ultrasound and although it's true that no long- or short-term problems have become apparent with it, it's being suggested that it has not been in use long enough to be totally sure of its harmlessness. The difficulty now is that so many women have had ultrasound, that proper trials comparing sufficiently large numbers of scanned babies and mothers with unscanned mothers and babies over a period of many years may be impossible.

UMBILICAL CORD This is the link between your baby and the placenta. It's greyish in colour and it measures about 60 centimetres (2 feet) in length. Inside are two arteries which carry 'used' blood back to the placenta, and one vein which carries fresh oxygenated blood back again to the fetus. The cord is clamped and cut shortly after birth, and the stump that's left drops off by itself in the first week or fortnight afterwards. Standard care of the cord stump is to keep it clean and dry before it drops off, and the midwife will check it daily to watch for infection (see *cutting the cord*).

URINARY TRACT INFECTION Not uncommon during pregnancy. It's any sort of infection that affects the tubes leading from the kidneys to the bladder (ureters). Hormonal effects on the ureters cause them to relax and they can be compressed by the uterus or kinked in some way. This causes the urine to stay in the ureters longer than it should, which increases the risks of infection. Symptoms are sickness, nausea, high temperature and pain. Antibiotics, plenty of fluids to flush out the infection, and rest, deal with the problem quickly and effectively.

URINATION You'll find you may need to pass water more often than usual in the first three months or so of pregnancy. This is thought to be because hormonal reaction causes your bladder and other tissues to be less taut, and so you feel the need to go to the lavatory more quickly. In the last couple of months or so, the uterus may press on your bladder, and this makes you feel the urge more often too. You may need to get up once or twice in the night (good practice for after the birth!).

During labour, the midwife will ask you to pass water every few hours so there's no chance of a full bladder holding up the progress of delivery. She also checks your urine for *protein* and *ketones*.

Normal healthy newborns pass water for the first time in the first two days, tell the midwife if your baby doesn't. Don't panic if you see a red stain on the nappy in the early days; again, check with the midwife, but it's most likely to be the baby getting rid of salts called urates, which have this staining effect.

URINE TEST You'll be asked to bring a urine sample to every ante-natal appointment and the staff will check it on the spot for *protein*, *sugar*, signs of infection and *ketones*. Bring your sample in a clean, well-rinsed container (you only need a small amount). The best 'catch' is from a mid-stream specimen. You begin to urinate, then catch an inch or so, and then continue in the lavatory. If you forget your sample, don't worry. You can always produce one at the clinic, and the staff will give you a jug or a basin.

UTERUS The womb. In a non-pregnant woman it's rather like an average size pear in both size and shape. It's hollow and joined at the top on either side to the *fallopian tubes*. The other end (the narrow part) finishes in the *cervix*, or the neck of the womb, which lies at the top of the vagina.

When a woman becomes pregnant, the fertilised egg embeds itself in the lining of the uterus. Hormonal action causes the uterus to

UTERUS

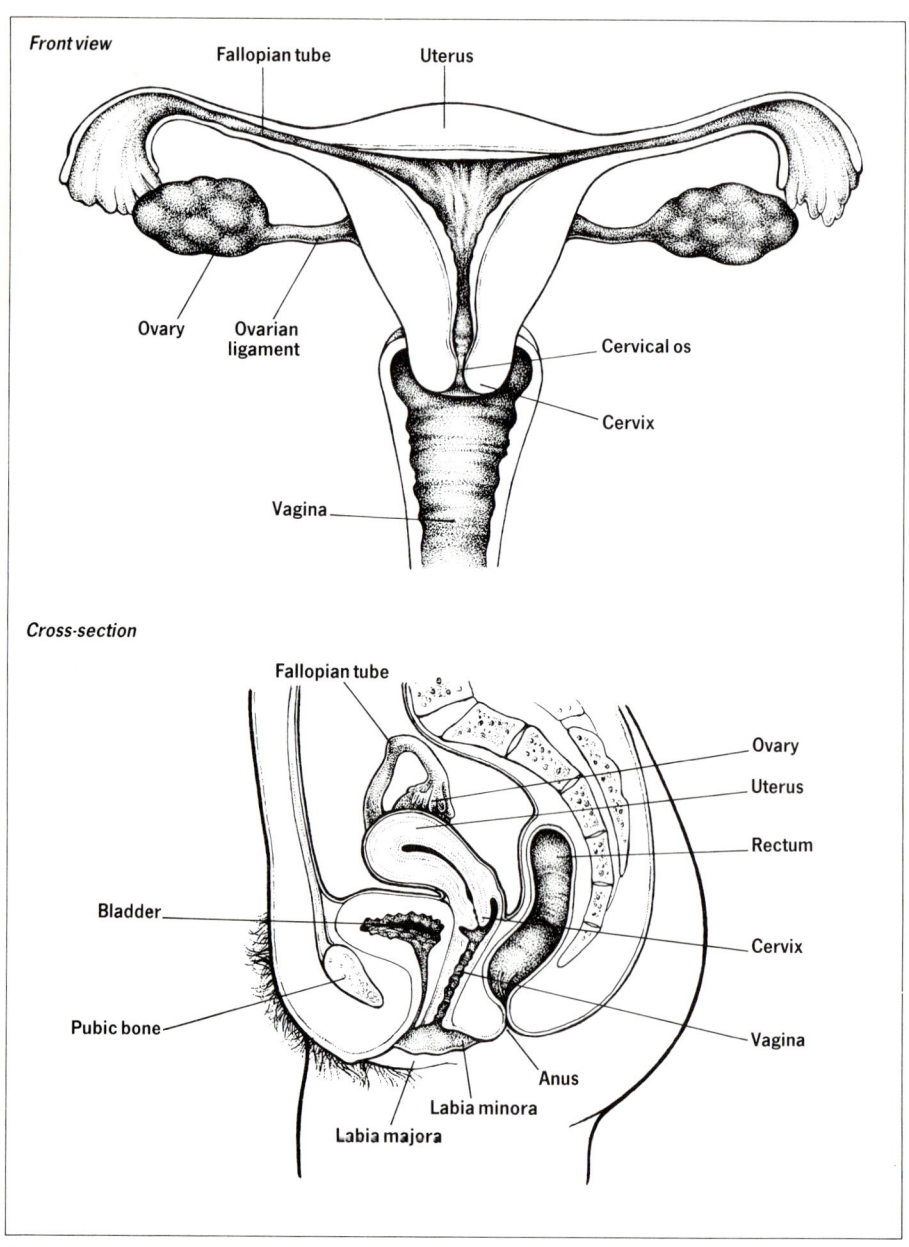

Front view

Cross-section

Reproductive organs

128

begin enlarging, and this continues throughout pregnancy to accommodate the growing fetus. The size of the uterus is regularly checked in pregnancy and its height is noted (the highest part of the uterus is called the fundus). It's one way of checking that your dates are accurate and that the baby is growing at the expected rate.

During labour, the uterus – which is formed of very many muscular fibres – contracts (you can mimic this action by tightening and loosening a clenched fist). This action of contracting very gradually pulls back the cervix to make the opening wide enough for the baby to pass through. At the same time it directs the baby downwards. The muscle fibres of the uterus become slightly shorter with each contraction, so there is less room in there for the baby. In the second stage, the contractions actively help to push the baby down through the birth canal and out. Further contractions expel the placenta in the third stage of labour.

Afterwards, the uterus is more like its non-pregnant size and shape, though it continues to contract for some days and even weeks. A uterus that's been pregnant is never exactly the same size, however, as it was.

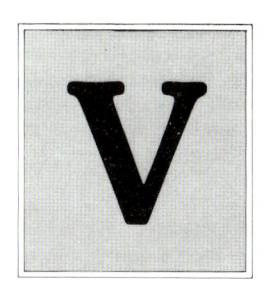

V-BAC An American term gaining slow currency in this country, meaning 'vaginal birth after caesarean'.

VACUUM EXTRACTION See *ventouse*.

VAGINA The internal passage, about 10 centimetres (4 inches) long, that leads from the vulva to the cervix. It becomes part of the birth canal when the baby is being delivered.

VAGINAL DISCHARGE It's quite normal for there to be some discharge from the vagina during pregnancy, and though it doesn't have the same sort of cyclical changes you may notice when you aren't pregnant, the amount can be more profuse than you are used to. Only if it appears smelly, coloured, or itchy is there any need to take medical advice (you could, for instance, have a vaginal infection such as *thrush*). After the baby is born you will have several days, perhaps weeks, of vaginal discharge known as *lochia*.

VARICOSE VEINS Varicose veins can appear during pregnancy, usually in the legs, as a result of slow blood circulation in the veins. It's possibly caused by the hormonal effects of pregnancy which soften and relax body tissue, including the walls of blood vessels. The veins appear swollen, and they

VENEREAL DISEASE

may ache maddeningly. The treatment is to wear support stockings or tights (stockings can be prescribed by your GP) and to give your legs a rest by putting your feet up at intervals during the day. Varicose veins can also appear in the vulva. Ask your doctor's or midwife's advice on dealing with the problem. A close-fitting sanitary pad can relieve the discomfort.

VENEREAL DISEASE The other name for STD – sexually transmitted diseases. Possibly dangerous for a baby: gonorrhea, for instance, can affect a baby during delivery, as the virus can make him blind. Syphylis can give the baby congenital syphylis. Most pregnant women's blood is routinely tested for venereal disease from a sample of blood taken when she books in for her delivery early in pregnancy. If you think you may have run the risk of contracting a venereal disease, then tell your doctor or ante-natal clinic. Or, simply, turn up at your local 'special clinic'.

VENTOUSE An alternative to *forceps*, used more abroad than in the UK, largely because of simple preference. It's formed of a metal cup, placed on the baby's scalp. A vacuum is created inside the cup, by using a small hand pump connected to the cup to suck the air out. This makes the cup adhere to the baby's scalp, and then the cup can be used to help the doctor guide the head down the birth canal. The vacuum is released after the birth, and the cup simply comes away from the scalp. It leaves a swelling called a *chignon*, which soon disappears (in a matter of hours). The process is also known as vacuum extraction.

VERNIX The full name for this is vernix caseosa. It's a greasy substance that comes from the baby's sebacious glands while he is still in the womb. It starts to appear at about 30 weeks and his body is well-covered with it by 36 weeks. It may still be there when he is born. The function of vernix is to protect the skin, insulate the baby and maybe to act as a sort of lubricant during the birth.

VITAMIN K This vitamin is used by the liver to make a protein necessary to prevent haemorrhage. In order to prevent a rare condition called haemorrhagic disease of the newborn some units give the majority of new babies a routine injection of vitamin K shortly after birth. You may see it noted as 'Konakion given' – Konakion is a brand name of manufactured vitamin K.

VITAMINS These are substances essential to life and health, found mainly in food. There are literally dozens of different vitamins, and for convenience they're given letter names. For example, vitamin C, vitamin B12 as well as their 'real' names ascorbic acid, riboflavin and so on. Certain vitamins need to be taken every day as the body cannot store them. Others are needed to convert vital food substances into forms the body can use. During pregnancy, and breastfeeding, the body's needs for vitamins A and D in particular increase. You can get vitamin A from milk, eggs, carrots, spinach, watercress and other green leafy vegetables, offal and oily fish. Vitamin D is in

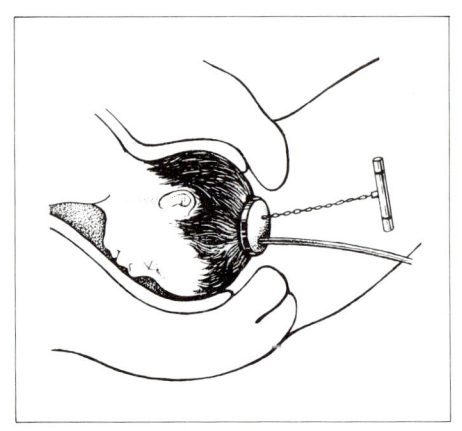

In order to help the birth of the baby's head, the ventouse is attached by gentle suction.

VULVA

similar animal sources as vitamin A, and margarine too (most margarine in the UK is fortified with vitamin D). The body can make its own vitamin D from sunlight, so it's a good idea to make sure you get out of doors on a sunny day.

VOMITING IN LABOUR Some women vomit in labour, often towards the end of the first stage, but it's usually over and done with quite quickly. Your senses can be quite acute in labour, and this is why a strong perfume, or the smell of stale cigarettes, for instance, can really make you retch. Some hospitals give you an antacid regularly throughout labour which may settle a queasy stomach. Its main function is to reduce the acid content of the stomach, so you run less risk of inhaling acid gastric juice under general anaesthetic if an emergency caesarean section is called for.

VOMITING IN PREGNANCY If you are suffering from pregnancy *sickness* you may actually vomit – and vomit often. If the measures suggested in this book don't help and your midwife or doctor have no other simple remedies to suggest, it may be necessary to seek further advice. This is because severe prolonged vomiting can affect your health and the health of your baby, as you can't keep any food down long enough for you and your baby to be nourished.

VULVA The external sexual organs of a woman.

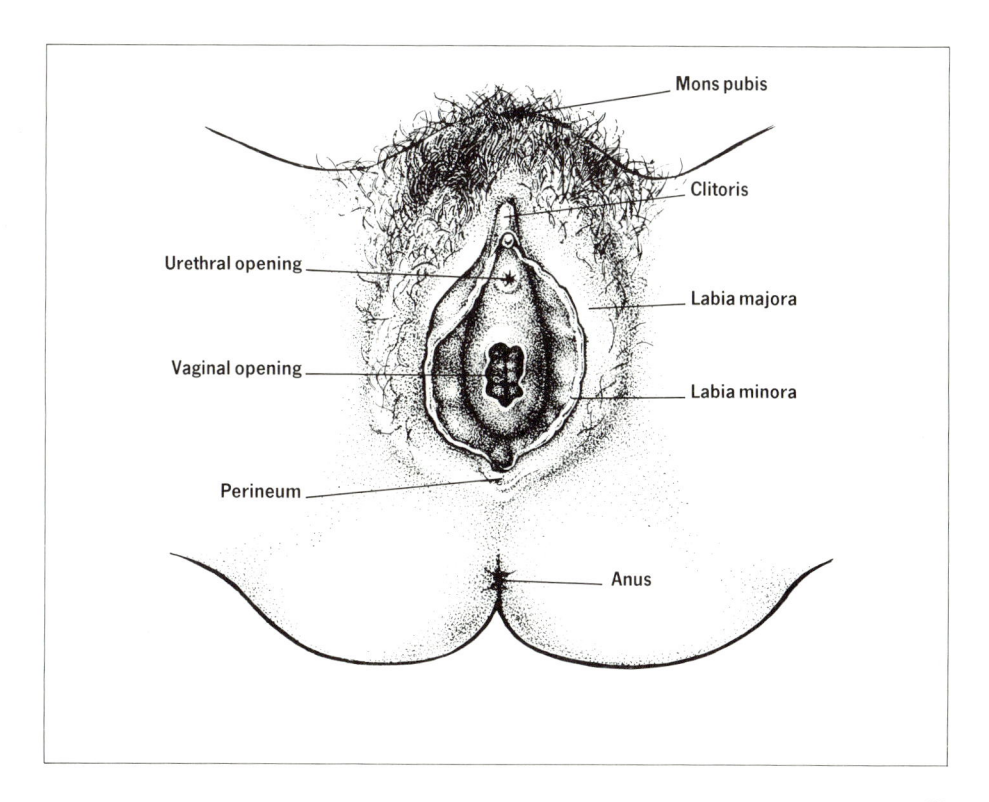

131

VULVAL HAEMATOMA A fortunately rare complication in the hours or days after birth. It happens when a vein (or veins) in the mother's vaginal ruptures, allowing blood to leak into the adjoining skin of the vulva and vaginal wall. It produces a painful swelling, and it needs prompt treatment, which is usually surgical. Under anaesthetic, the haematoma is drained to remove the blood.

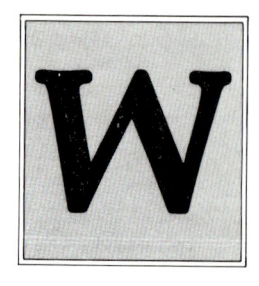

WASHING BABY See *topping and tailing*.

WATER RETENTION See *oedema*.

WATERS The *amniotic fluid* contained within the membranes in the uterus.

WEIGHING BABY Your baby's birth weight will be noted soon after she's born, and regular weighing afterwards helps to keep a check on her health, although there's less emphasis now on rigid weekly weight gains as 'proof' of health. Your baby will probably lose weight in the first week or so, and then she may take up to another couple of weeks to regain it (sometimes even longer). An obviously healthy baby only needs weighing once or twice a fortnight in her first few weeks, and much less frequently than this after that (see *weight gain of baby*).

WEIGHT GAIN OF BABY Experienced health visitors and midwives look at the baby before the weight gain chart. A healthy contented baby may not show the same rate of weight gain as her neighbour, but she could still be hale and hearty. These days, mothers are told much less frequently that their babies 'ought' to gain so much per week or per month. Individual variations are so wide that rules of thumb like these can be misleading; weight gain is only one of the factors used in assessing a baby's health. Nevertheless, a small and irregular weight gain over a few weeks needs to be taken seriously, even if all it means is that a baby's pattern is taking a while to settle down. A weight loss can be due to illness or underfeeding, too. In most cases of slow or worrying weight gain, a baby with problems will show other symptoms as well. If you're breastfeeding, and your baby doesn't seem to be gaining weight sufficiently well, or if the clinic is concerned about his weight, try feeding much more often. This will mean waking your baby, if she likes to sleep a lot. Extra rest and a good diet, plus extra feeding, usually does the trick. You should certainly do all this before you even think about complementary or supplementary bottles.

WEIGHT GAIN OF MOTHER The average weight gain during pregnancy is about 12.5 kilograms (28 pounds), although being an average, some women gain less and some gain more. There used to be a bit of a panic if you looked as if you were going to gain more than the average, partly because it can be a sign of *pre-eclampsia*, but also because it was thought it would hang about you as fat for the rest of your life. We now know this needn't be so. Some women just seem to gain a lot of weight quite naturally, and though they don't lose it all immediately, with a nutritious and sensible diet, the weight does eventually disappear. On the other hand women who gain very little weight in pregnancy are more likely to have small babies, and very small babies tend to have more problems at birth. The point is that eating the right sorts of foods in pregnancy is important to your health, and

WORK DURING PREGNANCY

WOMB See *uterus*.

WOOLWICH SHELLS See *breast shells; flat nipples; inverted nipples*.

WORK DURING PREGNANCY Your employer is not usually allowed to sack you simply because you're pregnant, and if you are in an unsuitable job for pregnancy he is obliged to try and find you alternative work. Unsuitable work would include anything involving a lot of bending or heavy lifting; contact with chemicals or dangerous substances; contact with X-rays. If you're in doubt, ask your doctor. You can also talk to your personnel department or union representative.

Lots of healthy women work until quite near the end of their pregnancy, but do consider whether you really have to. If you can claim maternity pay there's much less financial incentive to work right to the end. Who cares if you prove you're superwoman and go straight from the commuter train to the labour ward? A couple of months or so off work while you wait for your baby can be luxuriously restful, especially if it's your first, and the lack of stress at home can bring a peaceful frame of mind that's a real tonic! In the months and weeks before leaving work, make sure you avoid the usual pressures of rush and bustle if at all possible; have a quiet stroll outside in your lunch hour rather than the frantic dash round the shops most working women end up with. If it helps, see if you can negotiate some sort of flexi-time to help you avoid rush hours. And remember, you have a legal right to get paid time off to attend ante-natal clinics. If you want to find out more about your rights at work while you are pregnant, the Department of Employment issues a leaflet called 'Employment Rights for the Expectant Mother'. You can get this from your local Job Centre or Citizens' Advice Bureau, both of which will be able to help you if you have any other queries (see *maternity rights*).

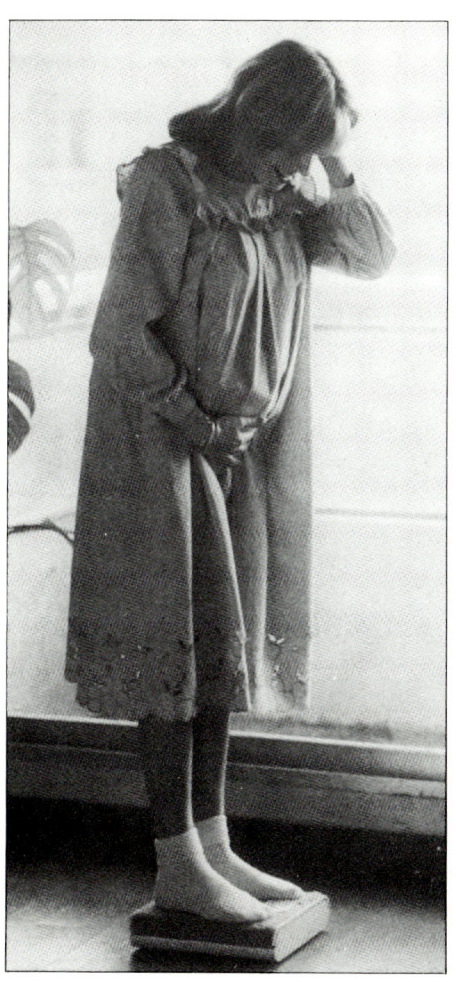

An erratic or slow weight gain isn't necessarily abnormal.

your baby's, and if you do this, you will probably gain something between 9 kilograms (20 pounds) and 15.5 kilograms (35 pounds). Any sudden weight gain or weight loss should be watched for; otherwise, eat well, eat normally, and don't worry.

133

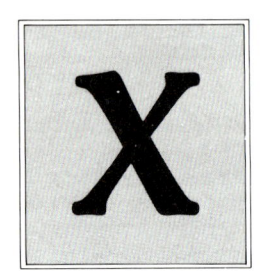

X-RAYS Electromagnetic waves that penetrate most substances. Until fairly recently X-rays were used in pregnancy for various diagnostic reasons. Now, because of the small risk of radiation affecting the baby, X-rays are done only when necessary. You may have one if it's thought there's a risk of *disproportion*.

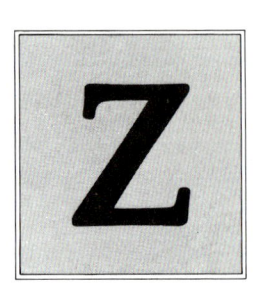

ZYGOTE When the egg is fertilised by a sperm, it is termed a zygote.

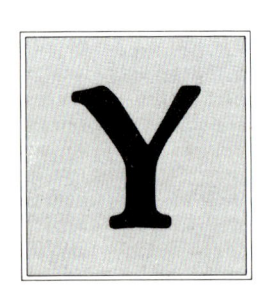

YELLOW SKIN Yellow skin in a newborn baby can mean he is jaundiced (see *jaundice*).

USEFUL ADDRESSES

THE ACTIVE BIRTH MOVEMENT
47 Pilgrim's Lane, London NW3
01-794 2354

Information on active birth, classes; teacher training

ASSOCIATION FOR IMPROVEMENTS IN THE MATERNITY SERVICES
163 Liverpool Road, London N1 0RF

Pressure group. Local branches plus newsletter

ASSOCIATION OF BREASTFEEDING MOTHERS
131 Mayow Road, London SE26
01-778 4769

For a recorded list of ABM counsellors

THE CAESAREAN SUPPORT NETWORK
c/o 11 Duke Street, Astley, Manchester M29 7BG

Information on local groups; leaflets

DOWNS CHILDREN'S ASSOCIATION
4 Oxford Street, London W1
01-580 0511/2

FAMILY PLANNING ASSOCIATION
27–35 Mortimer Street, London W1N 7RJ
01-636 7866

See your local telephone directory for nearest clinic

SOCIETY TO SUPPORT HOME CONFINEMENT
Lydgate House, Lydgate Lane, Wolsingham, Bishop Auckland, Durham DL13 4HA
0388 52 8044

Help and support for women wanting home birth. Leaflets available, SAE essential

FOUNDATION FOR THE STUDY OF INFANT DEATHS
5th floor, 4–5 Grosvenor Place, London SW1X 7HD
01-235 1721, 245 9421

Support and information for parents of cot-death victims

LA LECHE LEAGUE
BM 3424, London WC1N 3XX
01-404 5011

Breastfeeding advice. Local groups. International organisation

MATERNITY ALLIANCE
59-61 Camden High Street, London NW1
01-388 6337

Up to date information on maternity rights and benefits. Campaigns for a better deal for parents and children

NAWCH – THE NATIONAL ASSOCIATION FOR THE WELFARE OF CHILDREN IN HOSPITAL
Argyle House, 29–31 Euston Road, London NW1 2SD
01-833 2041

USEFUL ADDRESSES

NATIONAL CHILDBIRTH TRUST
9 Queensborough Terrace, London W2
01-221 3833

Ante-natal teaching; breastfeeding counselling; post natal groups nationwide

ASSOCIATION FOR POST NATAL ILLNESS
7 Gowan Avenue, London SW6

Information and support for women suffering from post-natal depression

SICKLE CELL SOCIETY
c/o Brent Community Health Council, 16 High Street, London NW10 4LX
01-451 3293

ASSOCIATION FOR SPINA BIFIDA & HYDROCEPHALUS
Tavistock House North, Tavistock Square, London WC1H 9HJ
01-388 1382

STILLBIRTHS & NEONATAL DEATHS ASSOCIATION (SANDS)
Argyle House, 29–31 Euston Road, London NW1 2SC
01-833 2851

Counselling and befriending for people who have lost a baby

TWINS AND MULTIPLE BIRTHS ASSOCIATION
c/o 292 Valley Road, Lillington, Leamington Spa, Warwickshire CV32 7UE

Leaflets, information and a network of local groups

TWINS CLUBS ASSOCIATION
Pooh Corner, 54 Broad Lane, Hampton, Middlesex TW12 3BG

For all parents of twins, triplets and more. Information, support and practical help

INDEX

A

abdomen 1
abortion 1, 5
  recurrent abortion 106
acceleration of labour 1, 10
active birth 1, 27, 92
acupuncture 2
adoption 2, 24
affiliation order 16
afterbirth *see* placenta
afterpains 2
age of mother 2
AID (artificial insemination by donor) 3
AIH (artificial insemination by husband) 3
alcohol 3, 38
allergies 3
all-fours, 2, 4, 18
alphafetoprotein 4
amenorrhoea 4
amniocentesis 4, 32, 46
amniotic fluid 4, 6, 64, 100
amniotic sac 6
anaemia 2, 20
anaesthetist 6, 51
analgesia 6 *see* pain relief
anencephaly 4, 6
ankles, swollen 6 *see* oedema
ante-natal care 6, 114
ante-natal classes 7, 98, 108, 164
ante-natal clinic 7, 8
ante-partum haemorrhage 5, 8, 19, 20
anterior lip of cervix 9
anterior presentation 9
antibodies 9, 24, 33, 65
anti-D gamma globulin 9, 65, 142
anxiety in labour 9
  in pregnancy 9, 50, 60
Apgar test 9
appearance of newborn 10
apnoea mattress 10
artificial rupture of membranes 1, 10, 75

aspirin 46
asthma 3

B

baby clinic 10, 64
backache 12
bath (in labour) 12
bathing baby 12
bearing down 12, 52, 97
bedding for baby 14
bedrest 14, 20
benefits *see* child benefit, maternity rights
bicornuate uterus 14
birth 14 and *passim*
birth certificate 16
birth chair 16
birth position 17
birthing room 16, 40
birthmarks 17
bladder 19
blastocyst 19, 42
bleeding 8, 14, 19, 31, 48, 49, 73
blighted ovum 19
blocked ducts 19, 24, 87
blood pressure 6, 14, 19
blood sugar level 36, 74
blood tests 20
blood transfusion 20
bloom of pregnancy 20
bonding 21
booking appointment 8, 22
bottle feeding 23, 60, 74
bouncing cradle 55
Braxton-Hicks contractions 24
bras 19, 23, 51
breastfeeding 2, 3, 24, 37, 41, 50, 58, 60, 61, 63, 78, 79, 82, 84, 86, 87
breast milk 4, 9, 24, 89
breast pumps 26, 56
breast shells 27, 63
breasts 23, 26
breathing 2, 27, 97
breathing (of baby) 28, 62, 76, 104, 108

breathlessness 28
breech 28, 53
brow presentation 29
butterfly mask 29

C

caesarean section 5, 8, 28, 29, 44, 46, 48, 53, 57, 122
calcium 30, 37, 103
caput 30, 64
care of new baby *see* bathing, breastfeeding, bottle feeding, equipment, nappies, washing baby, topping and tailing, weighing baby
carpal tunnel syndrome 30
cartiocography 30 *see* fetal monitor
castor oil 30
catheter 31
caul 31
cephalhaematoma 31
cephalic 31
cervix 9, 31
  ripening of 31
  incompetent 75, 114
cervical erosion 31
child benefit 31
chloasma 29, 32
chorion biopsy 5, 32
chorionic villii 73
chorionic gonadotrophin 32, 67
chromosomes, chromosomal disorders 5, 32, 65
circumcision 32
cleft lip/palate 32
clinic, ante-natal *see* ante-natal clinic
clinic, baby *see* baby clinic
clothes (for baby) 32
clothes (for mother) 88
coil 58
colostrum 26, 33, 62
community health council 33
community midwife 6, 7, 33, 44, 105 *see* midwife

137

INDEX

complications of pregnancy 34
conception 34, 36, 64
confinement 35
congenital 35
congenital dislocation of the hip 35
consultant 35, 72
contraception 23 see family planning
contraceptive pill see pill
contractions 2, 14, 24, 35, 50
controlled cord traction 120
constipation 35, 50, 61
convulsions 36
co-operation card 36
cord see umbilical cord
cord, prolapse of 28, 48
  cutting of 38
corpus luteum 36
cows milk 4
cramp 37
crowning 37
crying 37
cyst 37
cystitis 38

D

dating the pregnancy 38, 65
death in childbirth 39
decidua 39
deep transverse arrest 39, 64
delivery room 40
demand feeding 41
dental checks 41
development of fetus 41
dextrose 46, 65
diabetes 6, 43, 100
diaphragm 43
diaphragm (cap) 43, 58
diarrhoea 43
diet 35, 37, 43, 61, 63, 105, 115, 131
dilation and curettage 38
dilation of cervix 31, 36, 44, 48, 62
discharge (from hospital) 72
discharge (vaginal) 44, 129 see lochia
disposable nappies 92
disproportion 29, 44, 48
distress, fetal see fetal distress
diuretics 44
domino delivery 33, 45
doula 45
Down's syndrome 2, 5, 45
drip 46, 65
drugs 38, 44, 46
dysmature 85

E

eating in labour 46
eclampsia 47
ectopic pregnancy 47, 57
eczema 3
EDD/EDC 48, 39
effacement 48
embryo 48
emergency birth 48, 63
emergency caesarean section 29, 48
emergencies in labour 49
emergencies in pregnancy 48
emotions 49, 50
endometrium 50
energy spurt 50
enema 12, 43, 50
engagement of head 50
engorgement 19, 26, 51, 56
Entonox (gas and air) 6, 51
epidural 15, 28, 30, 51, 97
episiotomy 18, 53, 118
equipment for baby 54
erosion, cervical 31
exercise 55
expressing milk 19, 26, 56
external cephalic version 28

F

face presentation 57
fallopian tubes 34, 42, 47, 57
false labour 57
false pregnancy 57
family planning 43, 57 see cap, coil, pill
fathers 58, 80, 98
fear of childbirth 60
feeding 23, 24, 41, 60
fetal alcohol syndrome 3
fetal distress 1, 48, 49, 60
fetal heart see heart of fetus
fetal monitoring 15, 30, 52, 60, 68
fetal movements 61
fetus, development of 41
fibre 35, 61
first feed 61
first stage of labour 9, 62
fits 36
fixing see latching on
flat babies 62
flat nipples 63
fluid retention 6, 30, 63
folic acid 63
fontanelle 63
food in labour 46
forceps 16, 18, 28, 30, 40, 52, 53, 57, 63 see ventouse
forewaters 64

formula milk 4, 23
friends 64
FSH (follicle stimulating hormone) 64
fundus 65

G

gammaglobulin 65
gas and air see Entonox
gene 64
general anaesthetic 65
genetic counselling 65, 67
german measles see rubella
glucose drip 65
gown, hospital 72
GP 6, 65, 70
GP unit 65
grande multipara 69
grasp reflex 109
growth spurt 41
Guthrie test 66
gynaecologist 66

H

haematoma, vulval 131
haemoglobin 6, 20, 67
haemolytic disease 111
haemophilia 5
haemorrhage 67 see ante-partum haemorrhage, post-partum haemorrhage
hair 67
handicap 5, 67
HCG (Human chorionic gonadotrophin) 61, 67
head of baby 63, 67
headaches 68
health before pregnancy 68
health during pregnancy 68 see diet
health visitor 7, 10, 45, 65, 68
heart of fetus 68
heartburn 68
height of mother 69
heroin 46
herpes 69
high blood pressure see blood pressure
high risk 69
high tech 69
hip, congenital dislocation of 35
history, medical 57, 89
home birth 6, 63, 69
home help 70
hormones 70 see oestriol, oestrogens, oxytocin, progesterone, prolactin

138

INDEX

hospital 32, 70, 72
hospital nursery 72
hospital staff 72 see midwife
human placental lactogen 20
hydrocephaly/hydrocephalus 74
hygiene 74
hydatidiform mole 73
hypertension see blood pressure
hyperventilation 74
hypnosis 74
hypoglycaemia 36, 74
hypospadias 74

I

incompetent cervix 75
incontinence, stress 119
incubator 75
induction 10, 70, 75
infertility 76
insomnia 76
intensive care 76
intercourse 77 see sex
internal examination 77
inverted nipples 78
involution of uterus 78
iron 6, 63, 78
itching 78
IUD 58
IVF (in vitro fertilisation) 35

J

jaundice 76, 78

K

ketones, ketosis 47, 65, 79
kick chart 61, 79
Kitzinger, Sheila 103
kneeling 9, 18
Konakion 130
K, Vitamin 130

L

labour 80 and *passim*. See first stage of labour; second stage of labour; third stage of labour:
labour companion 80
labour, length of 82
labour, observations in 94
labour, signs of 116
labour ward 80
lactation see breastfeeding
lanugo 10, 42, 82

latching on 24, 26, 51, 63, 82, 117
laxatives 30, 35
Leboyer, Frederic 82
let-down reflex 84
lie of baby 84
light-for-dates 69, 85, 103
lightening 28, 84
linea nigra 85
liquor see amniotic fluid
lithotomy position 85
LH (luteinising hormone) 84
Local Health Council 33
lochia 19, 50, 86
loneliness 64
lungs, baby's 5, 42, 108

M

manual removal of placenta 86
massage 12, 86
mastitis 87
maternity rights 87
maternity wear 88
medical history 89
meconium 60, 89
membrane sweep 75
membranes 1, 6, 31, 89
mid-cavity arrest see deep transverse arrest
midwife 7, 33, 72, 89
milk see breast milk, cows milk, formula milk, soya milk
milk banks 89
miscarriage 1, 5, 19, 73, 75, 90, 121
menstruation see periods
mongolism see Down's syndrome
Montgomery's tubercles 26, 90
mother's age 2
Moro reflex 109
moulding 63, 90
movements, fetal 61
movement in labour 90
mucus extraction 90
mucus plug see show
multigravida 90
multipara 91

N

NAD 92
nappies 92
nappy changing 92
National Childbirth Trust 7, 32, 45, 64, 89
natural childbirth 92, 97
nausea 94
navel 94
neural tube defects 4, 5, 94
nipple shield 94

nipples, flat 63
inverted 78
notes 94
nursery 72

O

observations in labour 95
obstetrician 35, 94
occipito anterior 9
occipito posterior 39, 51, 95
occiput 95
Odent, Michel 2
oedema 6, 63, 95
oestriol 20, 95
oestriol tests 95
old wives' tales 96
oligohydramnios 6
operculum 96
orgasm 96
os 96
ovarian cyst 37
overbreathing 74
ovulation 34, 36, 58, 60, 97
oxygen 96
oxytocin 1, 2, 46, 75, 84, 96
oxytocin challenge tests 76

P

paediatrician 73
pain, pain relief 6, 27, 36, 51, 97 see active birth; breathing; Entonox; epidural; Pethidine; psychoprophylaxis; relaxation; TNS; trilene
palpation 97
panting 97
parentcraft 98
paternity leave 98
pelvic floor exercises 54, 56, 98
peri-natal death 98
perineum 98
periods 4, 58
pessaries 98
Pethidine 6, 98
phenylketonuria (PKU) 66, 99
piles 35, 99
pill, contraceptive 4, 39, 58, 99
placenta 2, 6, 20, 99
low-lying 86
manual removal of 86
praevia 9, 51, 99
retained 38, 110
trapped 121
placental abruption 9, 48, 100
placental insufficiency 100
polyhydramnios 6, 100

139

INDEX

port wine stains 17
positions *see* birth position
positions for first stage 1, 18, 100
post-mature 10, 76, 101
post-natal blues 50, 101
post-natal depression 49, 64, 81, 101, 102
post-natal examination 102
post-natal exercises 101
posterior position (of baby) 12, 40
post-term *see* post-mature
pre-conceptual care 68
pre-eclampsia 6, 20, 30, 60, 63, 103
pregnancy 103 and *passim*
   length of 82
   signs of 116
   weight gain during 132
   work during 133
premature baby *see* pre-term baby
prepping 12, 50, 103
pressure marks 16
pre-term babies 10, 24, 26, 28, 53, 89, 103, 108
primigravida 104
primipara 104
progesterone 104
prolactin 58, 104
prolapse of umbilical cord 28, 46
prolapse of uterus 54, 104
prostaglandin 75, 105
protein in diet 105
protein in urine 105
psychoprophylaxis 27, 105
pudendal block 105
puerperium 105

Q

quickening 61, 106

R

reflexes of baby *see* responses of newborn baby
registration of birth 16, 106
relationships 106 *see* fathers, friends, siblings
relaxation 2, 9, 27, 50, 68, 108
respiratory distress syndrome 28, 108
responses of newborn baby 108
rest 110
Rhesus factor, rhesus disease 9, 20, 111
rooming-in 112
rooting reflex 109
rubella 20, 38, 112
rupture of membranes *see* artificial

rupture of membranes, membranes

S

Savage, Wendy 113
second stage of labour 14, 16, 113
sex 58, 77, 113
sex of fetus 5, 32
scan *see* ultrasound
shared care *see* ante-natal care
shave 114
Shirodkar stitch 75, 114
SHO (senior house officer) 72
show 80, 114
siblings 114
sickle cell disease 20, 115
sickness 115, 131
skin in pregnancy 116
sleep after the birth 115
small-for-dates *see* light-for-dates
smear test 116
smoking 116
soft spots 63
soya milk 4
special care 21, 108, 117
speculum 77
sphygmomanometer 118
spina bifida 4, 118
spotting 118
spontaneous vaginal delivery 118
squatting 2, 18
STD (sexually transmitted diseases) 130
stepping response 109
sterilising 23
sticky eye 118
stillbirth 98, 100, 118
stitches 118
stork's beak marks 17
stranded beetle position 85
strawberry marks 17
stress incontinence 119
stretch and sweep 75
stretch marks 23, 119
sugar drip 46, 47
sugar in urine 119
sugar, low blood 36
suitcase for hospital 119
suppositories 50
surfactant 108
swimming 12, 55
syntocinon 96, 120
syntometrine 120

T

tear in perineum 120
teeth in pregnancy 120

telemetry 3
term 120
terry nappies 92
tests in pregnancy 4, 5, 8, 20, 23, 95, 127
thalassaemia 120
thalidomide 46
third stage of labour 99, 120
threatened miscarriage 121
thrombosis 121
thrush 46, 121
tights 88, 130
tiredness 121
TNS 121
topping and tailing 122
toxaemia *see* pre-eclampsia
tranquillisers 122
transition 122
transverse lie 122
trial of labour 44, 122
trial of scar 122
trilene 123
trimester 123
triplets 123
trophoblast 6, 123
twins 4, 82, 123
tubal pregnancy 47

U

ultrasound 5, 8, 39, 125
umbilical cord 127
   prolapse of 28, 48
   cutting of 38
urates 127
urinary tract infection 127
urination 127
urine, protein in 105
urine, sugar in 119
urine test 127
uterus 127
   bicornuate 14
   retroverted 110

V

vacuum extraction *see* ventouse
vagina 129
valium 47
varicose veins 129
V-Bac 129
venereal disease 20, 130
ventouse 64, 130
vernix 130
version, external cephalic 28
vitamins 130
Vitamin K 130
vomiting in labour 131

140

INDEX

vomiting in pregnancy 131
vulva 131
vulval haematoma 131

W

waters, breaking of 10 *see* amniotic fluid
weighing baby 132

weight gain of baby 131
weight gain of mother 131
Woolwich shells *see* breast shells
work during pregnancy 133

X

X-rays 38, 44, 134

Y

yellow skin 134 *see* jaundice
yoga 55

Z

zygote 134